ENTRANCE EXAMINATION IN TRANSFUSION MEDICINE

(Includes Important Text, Original Solved MCQs)

ENTRANCE EXAMINATION IN TRANSFUSION MEDICINE

(Includes Important Text, Original Solved MCQs)

Editor:

Dr. M.S. Bhatia
(M.D., MNAMS)
Prof. & Head, Department of Psychiatry
University College of Medical Sciences &
Guru Teg Bahadur Hospital
Dilshad Garden, Delhi-110095

Contributing Editor:

Dr. (Mrs.) Nirmaljit Kaur
(M.D.)
Senior Specialist, Department of Microbiology
Dr. Ram Manohar Lohia Hospital
New Delhi-110001

CBS

CBS PUBLISHERS & DISTRIBUTORS PVT. LTD.

NEW DELHI • BENGALURU • PUNE • KOCHI • CHENNAI

ISBN : 978-81-239-2185-3

First Edition : 2012

Published by Satish Kumar Jain and produced by V.K. Jain for
CBS Publishers & Distributors Pvt. Ltd.,
CBS Plaza, 4819/XI Prahlad Street, 24 Ansari Road, Daryaganj,
New Delhi - 110002, India. • Website: www.cbspd.com
e-mail: delhi@cbspd.com, cbspubs@airtelmail.in
Ph.: 23289259, 23266861, 23266867 • Fax: 011-23243014

Branches:

- ***Bengaluru:*** Seema House, 2975, 17th Cross, K.R. Road,
  Bansankari 2nd Stage, Bengaluru - 560070 Ph.: +91-80-26771678/79
  • E-mail: cbsbng@gmail.com, bangalore@cbspd.com
- ***Pune:*** Bhuruk Prestige, Sr. No. 52/12/2+1+3/2,
  Narhe, Haveli (Near Katraj-Dehu Road By-pass), Pune - 411051
  Ph.: +91-20-64704058/59, 32342277 • E-mail: pune@cbspd.com
- ***Kochi:*** 36/14, Kalluvilakam, Lissie Hospital Road,
  Kochi - 682018, Kerala • Ph.: +91-484-4059061-65
  Fax: +91-484-4059065 • E-mail: cochin@cbspd.com
- ***Chennai:*** 20, West Park Road, Shenoy Nagar, Chennai - 600030
  Ph.: +91-44-26260666, 26208620 E-mail: chennai@cbspd.com

Printed at :
J.S. Offset Printers, Delhi

Dedicated to our Parents

&

beloved Children

PREFACE

Medical science is a rapidly advancing field. Its new allied branches are coming up. In a competitive examination, more and more emphasis is being laid on these allied disciplines. But most of the standard textbooks of medicine have failed to devote adequate space to these new disciplines.

This book has been written with the aim to outline the major areas of Transfusion Medicine, a new superspeciality. This book is not merely an addition to the existing list of books on MCQ's but a sincere ambition and an honest attempt to make it a useful and practical companion to both medical graduates and postgraduates. The present book consists of original solved MCQ's from the *Question Banks* of various important examinations (AIIMS, Delhi, PGI etc.), Important text, original solved MCQ's have been added. We hope that this will help the candidates in performing better in the examination.

All suggestions for the modification of this book are welcome and will be duly acknowledged.

—Editors

CONTENTS

Preface *vii*

IMPORTANT TEXT 1—36

ORIGINAL MCQ's 39—75

MCQ's ASKED IN VARIOUS ENTRANCE EXAMS 79—111

GLOSSARY 115—142

ANNEXURE-I 145

ANNEXURE-II 146—147

IMPORTANT TEXT

IMPORTANT TEXT OF TRANSFUSION MEDICINE

* Volume of 1 unit of packed cells — 280 mls ± 60
* Fondaparinux is a synthetic pentasaccharide and potentials the action of antithrombin-III. It can be used in HITT (Heparin induced thrombocytopenia with or without thrombosis) patients.
* Blood is stored at -6°C
* Shelf life of blood is 35 days
* Platelets obtained and stored

  They are pooled 55×10^9

  1 adult dose = 240×10^9

  Stored at room temperature : -20 to -24°C

  Shelf half life is 7 days
* FFP should ideally be obtained of same ABO group. If it is not available, FFP of a different ABO group is acceptable because it does not possess anti- A and anti-B activity above a limit designated to detech high titres.
* HIT is Heparin induced thrombocytopenia (HIT) with or without thrombosis (HITT).

  It is seen with unfractioned heparin and typically 4-14 days after.
* *Type I* - is transient decrease in platelet count without any further symptoms. Count rarely goes below.

  Type II - is due to antiimmune reaction with antibodies formed against platelet factor 4 (PF4), neutrophil activating peptide 2 (NAP-2) and IL-B.
* Massive blood transfusion is defined as entire blood replaced within 24 hours (7% of body volume) or 50% in 3 hours (i.e > 10 units of red cells in 24 hours).
* Warfarin blocks post-ribosomal carboxylation of glutamic acid residues on factors II, VII, IX, X.
* Blood warming is contraindicated in massive transfusion.

* Depletion of coagulation factors usually occurs after 0.25 x blood volume has been lost.
* Beriflex is a prothrombin complex concentrates which can rapidly reverse the anticoagulant effect of heparin should occurs life threating bleeding.
* Hypercalcemia is complication of massive transfusion.

Autosomal Inheritance shows a characteristic pattern that is easy to recognize in both the dominant and recessive condition. The following are criteria for autosomal dominant inheritance.

1. The trait appears in every generation.
2. The trait occurs with equal frequency in males and females.
3. On the average, the trait is transmitted by an affected person to half of his or her children.
4. Unaffected family members do not transmit the trait to their children.

Most blood group antigens fit into this category. When two alleles are present, both traits are expressed and are said to be condominant. An autosomal recessive trait is expressed only in homozygotes who have received the recessive gene from both parents. The following are the criteria for autosomal recessive inheritance :

1. The trait characteristically appears only in siblings, not in the parents or other relatives.
2. On the average, one fourth of the siblings are affected.
3. The parents of the affected child may be consanguineous.
4. Males and females are equally likely to be affected.

Parents of affected children who lack the trait must necessarily be carriers, that is, heterozygous for the gene whose presence is not phenotypically apparent. When a recessive gene is rare, related persons are more likely to carry the same rare gene than are unrelated persons.

X-LINKED INHERITANCE

Dominant and recessive traits may be determined by genes on the X-chromosomes. When the gene products of sex (X) linked genes are studied in females. The phenotype or expression of dominant and recessive traits is the same as that for autosomal genes because females have two X-chromosomes. In contrast, males have one X-chromosome and one Y chromosome, and most of the genetic material on the X-chromosome in males does not have an analogous region on the Y-chromosome. Males are said to be hemizygous for the X- chromosome. As a result, the expression of X-linked genes that specify a dominant trait is effectively the same in males and females but is quite different for recessive traits. An X-linked recessive trait is expressed by all males who carry the gene but by females only if they are homozygous. Consequently, X-linked recessive diseases uch as hemophilia are almost entirely restricted to males.

The following's are the criteria for X-linked dominant inheritance :

1. Affected males transmit the trait to all their daughters and none of their sons.
2. Affected heterozygous females transmit the trait to half their children of either sex.
3. Affected homozygous femlaes transmit the trait to all their children.
4. In rare X-linked dominant disorders, females are more often affected but are usually heterozygous and have a variable, less severe expression.

An X-linked dominant trait in blood group genetics is the X- blood group.

The following are the criteria for X-linked recessive inheritance.

1. The incidence of the trait is much higher in males than in females.
2. The trait is transmitted from an affected male through all his daughters to, on the average, half of each of their sons.
3. The trait is never transmitted directly from father to son.
4. The trait is transmitted from a carrier female to one half of her daughters (carriers and one half of her sons (affected).

Hemophilia A is the classic example of an X-linked recessive disease.

NUMERICAL AND ALPHABETICAL DESIGNATIONS FOR THE RH BLOOD GROUP SYSTEM

Numerical *Numerical*	*Alphabetical* *Alphabetical*	*Numerical* *Numerical*	*Alphabetical* *Alphabetical*
Rh1	D	Rh9	C^x
Rh2	C	Rh10	V
Rh3	E	Rh11	E^w
Rh4	c	Rh12	G
Rh5	e	Rh13	Rh^A
Rh6	cis ce	Rh14	Rh^B
Rh7	cis Ce	Rh14	Rh^B
Rh8	C^w	Rh15	Rh^c

(Contd....)

Numerical Numerical	*Alphabetical Alphabetical*	*Numerical Numerical*	*Alphabetical Alphabetical*
Rh16	RhD	Rh33	R^N Har
Rh17	Hr	Rh34	total Batiaan
Rh18	Hr	Rh35	RN-like
Rh19	hr	Rh36	Be
Rh20	VS	Rh37	Evans
Rh21	CG	+	+
Rh22	cis CE	Rh39	C and Hr-like
Rh23	Dw	Rh40	Tar
Rh24	E^T	Rh41	Ce-like
Rh26	c-like	Rh42	hr^H like
Rh27	cis cE	Rh43	crawford
Rh28	hr^H	Rh44	Nou
Rh29	"total Rh"	Rh45	Riv
Rh30	Go	Rh46	Sec
Rh31	hr^B	Rh47	Dav
Rh32	R^N	Rh48	JAL

TIPPETT'S GENETIC MODEL APPLIED TO THE EIGHT COMMON Rh GENE COMPLEXES

First Locus	*Second Locus*	*Gene Complex*	*Shorthand Symbol*
D	ce	Dce	R^0
D	Ce	DCe	R^1
D	cE	DcE	R^2
D	CE	DCE	R^Z
non-D	ce	dce	r
non-D	Ce	dCe	r'
non-D	cE	dcE	r"
non-D	CE	dCE	r^y

DIFFERENCE OF CLASS I AND CLASS II

	Class-I	*Class-II*
Antigens	HLA-A-,-B-,C	HLA-DR,-DP,-DO
Distribution	All nucleated cells, Platelets	B-lymphocytes Monocytes Macrophages Activated T-cells
Structure	Large polypeptide Chain (MHC coded) and a beta-2 Microglulin	Two polypeptide chains (alpha and beta) both MHC coded
Interacts	CD8 lymphocytes	CD4 lymphocytes. Mixed lymphocyte reaction

NORMAL VALUES OF RBC COUNT

Men	$5.5 \pm 1.0 \times 10^{12}/L$
Women	$4.8 \pm 1.0 \times 10^{12}/L$
Infants (full term cord blood)	$5.0 \pm 1.0 \times 10^{12}/L$
Children 3 months	$4.0 \pm 1.0 \times 10^{12}/L$
Children 1 year	$4.4 \pm 1.8 \times 10^{12}/L$
Children 3-6 years	$4.8 \pm 1.7 \times 10^{12}/L$
Children 10-12 years	$4.7 \pm 1.7 \times 10^{12}/L$

NORMAL VALUES

	MCV (ft)	*MCH (pg)*	*MCHC*
Normal adult	90 ± 10	31 ± 4	34 ± 3
Normal newborn	119 ± 9.0	36 ± 2	32 ± 3.2
Ages 10-17 months	77 ± 7	26.1 ± 2.8	34.2 ± 1.6
18-48 months	80 ± 6	27.0 ± 3.0	33.6 ± 1.4
4-7 years	81± 5	27.6 ±2.4	33.6 ±1.6

CONDITONS ACCOMPANIED BY ABNORMAL WHITE CELL COUNTS

High White Cell Count (leucocytosis)	*Low White Cell Count (leucopenia)*
Appendicitis	Measles
Pneumonia	Influenza
Leukemia	Brucellosis
Tonsillitis	Typhoid fever
Meningitis	Agranulocytosis
Abscesses	Infectious hepatitis
Rheumatic fever	Lupus erythematosus
Diphtheria	Cirrhosis of liver
Smallpox	Paratyphoid fever
Chickenpox	Protein therapy
Peritonitis	Radiation
Erythroblastosis fetalis	Myxedema
Uremia	Psittacosis
Ulcers	Sandfly fever
Newborn	Scrub typhus
Pregnancy	Dengue
Menstruation	Rheumatoid arthritis

ANTI-C, ANTI-C, ANTI-E AND ANTI-E ARE OCCASIONALLY SEEN AND MAY CAUSE BOTH TRANSFUSION REACTIONS AND HAEMOLYTIC DISEASE OF THE NEW-BORN. ANTI-D DOES NOT EXIST

CDE nomenclature	*Short symbol*	*RhD status*
cde/cde	r r	Negative
CDe/CDe	R_1 r	Positive
CDe/CDe	R_1R_1	Positive
cDE/cde	R_2 r	Positive
CDe/cDE	R_1R_2	Positive
cDE/cDE	R_2R_2	Positive
Other genotypes		Positive (almost all)

ABO BLOOD GROUP SYSTEM

Blood group Phenotype	*Genotype*	*Red cell Antigens*	*Naturally occurring antibodies*
O	OO	O	Anti-A, Anti-B
A	AA or AO	A	Anti-B
B	BB or BO	B	Anti-A
AB	AB	AB	None

THE DESIGNATIONS EMPLOYED BY THE TWO SYSTEMS FOR THE DIFFERENT RH TYPES ARE AS FOLLOWS

	Fisher	*Wiener*
Rh positive	CDe	Rh_1
	cDE	Rh_2
	cDe	Rh_0
	CDE	Rh_7
Rh negative	Cde	rh
	cdE	rh
	cde	rh
	CdE	rh

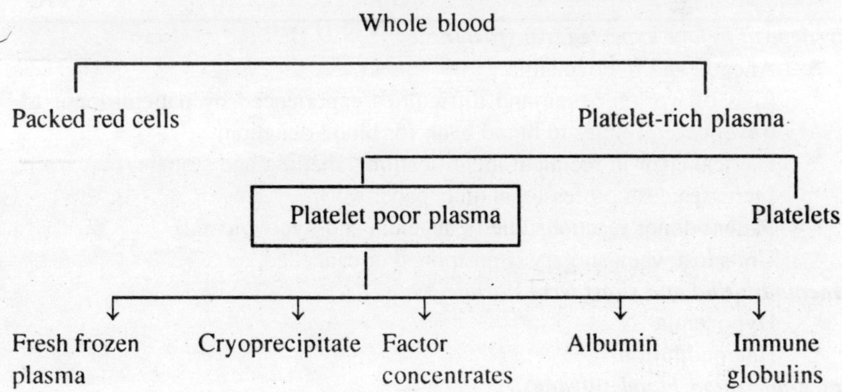

COMPLICATIONS OF BLOOD TRANSFUSION

Early	*Late*
Haemolytic reactions	Transmission of
Immediate	diseases e.g.
Delayed	Virus
Reactions due to	hepatitis A,B,C and others
Allergic reactions to	HIV
white cells, platelets	CMV
or proteins	Bacteria
Pyrogenic reactions	Treponema pallidum
(to plasma proteins	Brucella
or due to HLA	Salmonella
antibodies)	Parasites
Circulatory overload	Malaria
Air embolism	Toxoplasma
Thrombophlebitis	Microfilaria
Citrate toxicity	Transfusional iron
Hyperkalaemia	overload
Clotting abnormalities	Immune sensitization,
(after massive	e.g to RhD
transfusion)	antigen

CMV = Cytomegalovirus; HIV = Human Immunodeficiency Virus; HLA = human Leucocyte antigen.

HAZARDS OF AUTOLOGOUS TRANSFUSION

Predeposit before expected transfusion

* Anemia and hypovolemia.
* Loss of working time and difficulties experienced by patient-donor to travel several times to blood bank for blood donation.
* Clerical error in recipient identification, labelling and storage.
* Increased cost, professional time, paper work.
* Patient-donor reactions due to anaemia and hypovolemia.
* Units lost when surgery is postponed or cancelled..

Haemodilution and short term storage

* Hypoxemia
* Haemodilution

Intra-operation blood salvage

* Consumption of coagulation factor and platelets.
* Sepsis from contaminated blood.
* Cancer dissemination.

THE CHOICE OF ALTERNATIVE BLOOD

Patient's Blood Group	*Alternative Blood Group*	
	First Choice	*Second Choice*
A	O	None
A_2 with anti-A_1	O	None
A_1 with anti-HI(O)	None	None
B	O	None
A_1B	A or B	O
A_1B with anti-HI(O)	A_1 or B	None
A_2B	A or B	O
A_2B with Anti-A_1	A_2 or B	O

SELECTION OF ABO BLOOD GROUP FOR EXCHANGE TRANSFUSION IN Rh-HDN

Baby's blood group	*Mother's blood group*	*Blood selected for exchange transfusion*
A	A	A or O
	B	O
	AB	A or O
	O	O
B	A	O
	B	B or O
	AB	B or O
O	O	O
AB	A	A or O
	B	B or O
	AB	AB, A, B, O
	O	O
O	A	O
	B	O
	A,B	O
	O	O

ABO TYPING DISCREPANCIES

Weak reacting or missing antigens
- * ABO subgroups
- * Pathologic causes
- * Chimerism
  - Temporary
  - Genetic

Weak reacting or missing antibodies
- * Newborn
- * Pathologic causes
- * Chimerism
  - Temporary
  - Genetic
- * Prozoning
- * Elderly
- * ABO subgroups

Unexpected antigen reactions
- * Rouleaux
- * Antibody-coated red cells
- * Polyagglutination
- * Acquired B
- * Overlapping glycosyltransferase activity
- * In vitro immune complex attachment
- * Contaminating antibody in reagent
- * Agent causing nonspecific agglutination

Unexpected antibody reactions
- * Rouleaux
- * A subgroup with anti-A,
- * Cold autoantibodies
- * Cold alloantibodies
- * Passively acquired anti-A or anti-B

RESOLVING ABO TYPING DISCREPANCIES AND OTHER TYPING PROBLEMS

Testing blood from blacks with anti-e. A variant status should be investigated when alloantibody of apparent anti-e specificity is found in the serum of an e+ person, when a negative test result is obtained on testing a sample expected to be e+ with anti-e. or when discrepant results are observed when using more than one anti-e serum.

Antigen Typing Technical Errors

Technical errors can be due to clerical error, reagent/equipment dysfunction, or procedural error. The potential sources of error listed are essentially the same as those given for ABO discrepancies. The importance of adhering to the manufacturer's directions and using the appropriate control for the test system used cannot be overemphasized.

Antigen Typing Technical Errors are :

Clerical Errors

Sample identification

Test tubes mislabelled

Error in recording results

Reagent/Equipment dysfunction

Improper storage of reagents

Contaminated reagents

Incorrect centrifugation of tests

Procedural efforts

Failure to follow manufacturer's directions

Reagents not added to test

Use of the wrong reagent

Failure to use appropriate control for test

Misinterpretation of result

ACUTE ADVERSE EFFECTS OF TRANSFUSION

IMMUNOLOGIC

Hemolytic Transfusion Reactions

Mediators : IgM antibodies (Usually ABO), complement

Signs/symptoms : Fever, chills, hemoglobinemia, hemoglobinuria, hypotension, dyspnea

Management/prevention : Decrease opportunities for error, treat acute renal failure and DIC

Non-hemolytic Febrile Transfusion Reactions

Mediators antibodies to HLA Class-I antigens

Signs/symptoms : Fever, chills

Management/preventions : Antipyretics, leukocyte depletion

Allergic Transfusion Reactions

Mediators : Plasma proteins (mild reactions)-antibodies to IgA (anaphylactic reactions)

Signs/symptoms : Urticaria, erythemia, itching, anaphylaxis

Management/prevention : Antihistamines treat symptoms transfuse IgA deficient components

Non-cardiogenic Pulmonary Transfusion Reactions

Mediators : Donor/recipient white blood cell antibodies

Signs/symptoms : Acute respiratory distress, fever, chills, cyanosis, hypotension, noncardiogenic pulmonary edema

Management/prevention vigorous respiratory support steroids

Non-immunologic

Bacterial contamination

Mediators : Endotoxins produced by gram-negative bacteria

Signs/symptoms : Fever, shock, hemoglobinuria

Management/prevention : Intravenous antibiotics, treat, hypotension and DIC

Circulatory Overload

Mediators : Fluid volume

Signs/symptoms : Coughing cyanosis, orthopnea, severe headache peripheral edemy difficulty breathing

DELAYED ADVERSE EFFECTS OF TRANSFUSION

IMMUNOLOGIC

Hemolytic Transfusion Reactions

Mediator : IgG antibodies

Signs/symptoms : Shortened red blood cell survival, decreased hemoglobin, fever, jaundice, hemoglobinuria

Management/prevention : Antigen-negative blood for further transfusions

Transfusion-Associated Graft-versus-host disease

Mediators : viable donor lymphocytes

Signs/symptoms : Fever, skin rash, desquamation, anorexia, nausea, vomiting, diarrhea, hepatitis, pancytopenia

Management/prevention: Gamma irradiation of cellular components

(Contd.....)

DELAYED ADVERSE EFFECTS OF TRANSFUSION (Contd....)

Post-transfusion Purpura

Mediators : Platelet-specific antibodies

Signs/symptoms : Thrombocytopenia, clinical bleeding

Management/prevention: Intravenous immunoglobulins, plasma exchange, corticosteroids

NON-IMMUNOLOGIC

Transfusion-induced Hemosiderosis

Mediator : Iron overload

Signs/symptoms : Subclinical to death

Management/prevention : Decrease frequency of transfusions, neocytes, iron chelation therapy

POSSIBLE ADVERSE PHYSIOLOGIC CONSEQUENCES OF MASSIVE TRANSFUSION

Dilutional thrombocytopenia

Dilutional coagulopathy

Shift to left in oxygen-dissociation curve

Acid-base imbalance

Citrate toxicity

Hypothermia

Immunosuppression

Potassium overload

Respiratory distress

CLINICAL FEATURES ASSOCIATED WITH HYPOTHERMIA

Decreased metabolism of citrate and lactate

Decreased ability to regenerate 2,3-DPG

Platelet dysfunction

Impaired drug metabolism

Increased blood viscosity

Impaired hemostatic function

Acidosis

Hypoperfusion

Cardiac arrhythmias

CONDITIONS FOR WHICH PLASMA EXCHANGE IS INDICATED

Paraproteinemias
- Multiple myeloma
- Macroglobulinemia
- Cryoglobulinemia
- Pyroglobulinemia
- Connective tissue disease

Renal diseases
- Good pasture's syndrome
- Glomerulonephritis
- Renal transplant rejection

Familial hypercholesterolemia

Microangiopathic hemolytic anemia (TTP)

Immune complex diseases
- Systemic lupus erythematosus
- Rheumatoid arthritis
- Autoimmune hemolytic anemia

Neurologic disorders
- Guillain-Barre syndrome
- Myasthenia gravis
- Multiple sclerosis
- Eaton-Lambert syndrome
- Polymyositis

SOME CONDITIONS FOR WHICH THERAPEUTIC CYTAPHERESIS IS INDICATED

Plateletpheresis (thrombocytapheresis)
- Thrombocytosis (thrombotic or hemorrhagic)

Leukocytapheresis
- Leukemia (with hyperleukocytosis)
- Cutaneous T-cell lymphoma
- Hairy cell leukemia
- Collection of stem cells

Erythrocytapheresis
- Sickle cell anemia (with vaso-occlusion)

Lymphocytapheresis
- Rheumatoid arthritis

FEDERALAGENCIES WITH SAFETY REGULATIONS FORGUIDELINES

- Centers for Disease Control (CDC)
- Food and Drug Administration (FDA)
- Department of Transportation (DOT)
- Environmental Protection Agency (EPA)
- Nuclear Regulatory Commission (NRC)

SOME DRUGS ASSOCIATED WITH A POSITIVE DATE AND PROBABLE RED CELL DESTRUCTION

Drug Adsorption Autoimmune Hemolytic Anemia

Penicillin G
Methicillin
Nafcillin
Tetracycline
Cephalothin
Erythromycin
Carbromal
Cefazolin
Cefamandole
Cefotaxime
Cefotetan
Acetaminophen
Chlorpropamide

Methyldopa
Mefenamic acid
Levodopa
Procainamide

Immune Complex

Quinine
Quinidine
Phenacetin

Membrane modification

Cephalothin
Cisplatin
Diglycoaldehyde

Melphalan
Methotrexate
Rifampicin
Stibophen
Thiopental
Cefotaxime
Ceftriaxone

AGENCIES WITH VOLUNTARY GUIDELINES

National Committee on Clinical Laboratory Standards (NCCLS)
College of American Pathologists (CAP)
Joint Commission on Accreditation of Healthcare Organizations (JCAHO)
National Fire Protection Association (NFPA)

GENOTYPES AND PHENOTYPES IN ABO SYSTEM IN INDIAN POPULATION

Genotype	*Phenotype (Blood group)*	*Approx. Population (Percent)*
OO	O	40
AA AO	A2 A	2
BB BO	B B	33
AB	AB	5

* 93% of Indian population is Rh positive as compared to 85% in Northern Europe and North America.

BLOOD CELLS IN THALASSEMIA MAJOR, THALASSEMIA MINOR, AND IRON DEFICIENCY ANAEMIA

	Thalassemia major	*Thalassemia minor*	*Iron deficiency anaemia*
Peripheral blood			
Anisocytosis	2 - 4 +	1 - 2 +	1 - 2 +
Hypochronic Microcytosis	2- 4 +	1 - 3 +	2 - 4 +
Poikilocytosis	2 - 4 +	1 - 2 +	0 - 1 +
Polychromasia basophilic stippling	2 - 3 +	1 - 2 +	No
Target cells	3 - 4 +	2 - 3 +	0 - 1 +
Howell-jolly bodies	Occasional	No	No
Normoblasts	Occasional	Seldom	Seldom
Reticulocytes	Significantly increased	Moderately increased	Decreased to normal
Platelets	Normal to increased	Normal	Normal increased or decreased
White blood cells	Normal to increased	Normal	Normal to decreased
Bone marrow			
Erythroid hyperplasia	3 - 4 +	Normal to 2+	3 - 4 +
Haemosiderin	3 - 4 +	Normal to 2+	Absent

CELL DISTRIBUTION IN BONE MARROW AND PERIPHERAL BLOOD

Types of cells	*Marrow%*		*Peripheral blood%*	
	Average	*Range*	*Average*	*Range*
Myeloblasts	2.5	0.5-5	0	
Promyelocytes	6	1 - 8	0	
Myelocytes	15	8 - 20	0	
Neutrophilic	12	5 - 19	0	
Eosinophilic	1.5	0.5-3.0	0	
Basophilic	0.3	00 - 0.3	0	
Metamyelocytes	29	14 - 36	0	
Neutrophilic	26.4	13 - 32.0	0	
Eosinophilic	2.0	0.5 - 3.0	0	
Basophilic	2.0	0.5 - 3.0	0	
Segmented granulocytes	32	17 - 43		
Neutrophilic	27	15-35	60	50-70
Eosinophils	4	1 -7	2	1-4
Basophilic	1	0.5-1.5	0	0-1
Monocytes	2	04 - 4.0	5	2-10
Lymphocytes	13	5 - 20	30	2- - 40
Pronormoblasts	0.6	0.2 - 4	0	
Early normoblasts	2.4	1.5 - 5.8	0	
Intermediate normoblast	10.0	5.0 - 20.0	0	

(Contd....)

CELL DISTRIBUTION IN BONE MARROW AND PERIPHERAL BLOOD (CONTD.....)

Types of cells	Marrow% Average	Peripheral blood% Range	Average	Range
Late normoblast	6.6	3.0 - 20.0	0	
Megaloblasts	0.2	0 -0.5	0	
Megakaryocytes	0.5	0.04 - 2.0	0	
Reticulum cells	1.0	0.2 -3.0	0	
Plasma cells	0.6	0 - 2.0	0	
M : E Ratio	3-4 : 1			

SOME CLINICALLY IMPORTANT BLOOD GROUP SYSTEMS

Systems	Antigen	Frequency of antibodies	Causes of haemolytic transfusion reaction	Causes of haemolytic disease of newborn
ABO	AB (H-sustance)	Very common	Yes (common)	Yes
Rhesus	C c DEe	Common	Yes (common)	Yes
Kell	K k	Occasional	Yes (occasional)	Yes
Lewis	Lea Leb	Occasional	Yes (rare)	No
P	P1PPk	Occasional	Yes (rare)	Yes (rare)
I	Ii	Rare	Unlikely	No
Lutheran	Lua Lub	Rare	Yes (rare)	No
Duffy	Fya Fyb	Occasional	Yes (occasional)	Yes
Kidd	JKa JKb	Occasional	Yes (occasional)	Yes
MNSs	M N Ss	Rare	Yes (rare)	Yes (rare)

THE MORE SIGNIFICANT BONE MARROW ABNORMALITIES IN VARIOUS DISEASE

Disease	*Abnormality*	*Normal Values*
Aplastic anaemia	Hypoplastic (defective and incomplete development of cells)	Normoblastic
Iron deficiency anaemia	Hyperplastic (overactive); increase in nucleated red cells (30-60%)	Normoblastic
Pernicious anaemia	Increase in nucleated red cells (30-50%): presence of "pernicious anemia type" nucleated red cells	8- 30%
Hereditary spherocytic anaemias	Increase in nucleated red cells (30-60%)	8 - 30%
Sickle [illegible] anaemia	Increase in nucleated red cells (40 - 70%)	8 - 30%
Thalassemia major	Increase in nucleated red cells (30 - 60%)	8 - 30%
Acute granulocytic leukemia	Increase in myeloblasts (150 - 50%)	0 - 5%
Chronic granulocytic leukemia	Increase in myeloblasts (5 - 15%) increase in myelocytes and metamyelocytes	0.5%
Acute lymphocytic leukemia	Increase in lymphoblasts (15 - 75%)	0%
Chronic Gymplocytic leukemia	Increase in lymphocytes (30 - 90%)	5 - 15%
Monocytic leukemia	Increase in monocytes (20 - 60%)	0 - 5%
Plasmacytic leukemia	Increase in plasmacytes (15 - 75%)	0 - 1%
Purpura hemorrhagica (idiopathic thrombocy topenic purpura)	Number of megakaryocytes is normal or increased platelet formation is decreased	0 - 3%
Polycythemia vera	Hyperplastic; percentage normoblastic of white cells, red cells and platelets is normal	

THE MORE SIGNIFICANT BONE MARROW ABNORMALITIES IN VARIOUS DISEASE (Contd.)

Disease	*Abnormality*	*Normal Values*
Agranulocytosis	Granulocytes are decreased during height of disease but increased during recovery: percentage of nucleated red cells is normal	8 - 30%
	Percentage of megakaryocytes is normal	0 - 3%
Infectious mononucleosis	Increase in lymphocytes (15 - 35%)	5 - 15%
Multiple myeloma	10 - 90%	0%
Hodgkin's disease	Presence of Sternberg-Red cells	0%
Gaucher's disease	Presence of Gaucher's cells	0%

ANTIBODY DETECTION OR IDENTIFICATION ENHANCEMENT

Procedure	*Action*	*Effect*
Saline technique	High ions, low zeta potential	Basic conditions for antigen-antibody reactions
Albumin technique	Reduces dielectric constant and ion cloud	Enhances agglutination
LISS technique	Reduces concentration of ions, increases zeta potential	Increases speed of reaction, enhances sensitization
Enzyme technique	Removes sialic acid and proteins, decreases zeta potential, water of hydration, and ion cloud	Enhances sensitization and agglutination with many antibodies (esp. Rh and Kidd). While dena turing others (MNS blood group antigens, Duffy, and so forth)
Increase volume of serum	Increases number of antibody molecules	Increases sensitization, especially with high-affinity, low titer antibodies
Lengthen incubation time	Reaction approaches equilibrium	Increases sensitization
Vary temperature	Increases association of decreases dissociation rates	Optimum reaction conditions (e.g. anti-M at 16°C)
Selected homozygous red cells	Increased number of antigen sites per red blood cell	Increases sensitization
Add complement	Supplies complement	Increases polyspecific or anti-C AHG reactivity
Dilute serum	Dilutes antibodies or other proteins	Overcomes prozone and rouleaux
Change pH	Increases association or decreases dissociation rates	Increases reactivity with some antibodies
Absorb and elute into smaller volume or	Concentrates antibody concentrate serum	Increases sensitization

ELIMINATION OF ANTIGEN-ANTIBODY REACTIVITY

Procedure	*Action*	*Effect*
Prewarmed AHG test	By-passes cold auto or alloantibodies	Eliminates carry-over of cold into AHG phase
Anti-IgG AHG	By-passes complement activation	Eliminates complement carry-over of cold agglutinins
Enzymes	Inactivate antigens (e.g. Duffy, MNS)	Makes functional antigen-negative cells
AET or ZZAP	Destroys Kell antigens	Makes functional K cells
Sulfydryl treatment of serum	Denatures IgM immunoglobulins	Eliminates direct agglutination and complement activation by IgM globulins
Different media : LISS, saline, albumin	Uses different additives and preservatives	By-passes rouleaux, cold agglutinins, antibody reagent (e.g. caprylate, dye)
Increased temperature	Decreases association rates or increases dissociation rates	Eliminates cold-reactive antibodies
Decreased incubation time	Decreases sensitization	Decreases reactivity of cold agglutinins
Inhibition with specific substances	Neutralizes antibody	Eliminates anti-A, B, -Le, Leb, P1, Sd, Ch, Rg
Change in pH	Increases dissociation or decreases association rates	Eliminates some anti-M by pH
Saline replacement	Removes abnormal proteins	By-passes rouleaux
Washing of reagent red cells	Removes additives	By-passes reagent antibodies
No washing of red cells	Neutralizes antibody	Inhibits antibodies (e.g. anti-Ch, antiglucose)
Absorptions	Removes unwanted antibody(ies)	Eliminates
Cold auto		Cold agglutinins
Warm auto		Warm autoantibodies
Selected red cells		Alloantibodies or autoantibodies
Auto cells +C4		Anti-Ch and anti Rg
Platelets		Human lymphocyte antigen antibodies
Rabbit red cells		Anti-I, IH

INDICATIONS AND CONTRAINDICATIONS OF BLOOD AND BLOOD PRODUCTS

Blood and Blood Components	Indications for use	Contraindications for use
Whole blood (WB)	Restore/maintain blood volume and red cell mass in acute, massive blood loss	Volume replacement Correct anemia in normovolemic patients
Red blood cells (RBCs)	Increase red cell mass of symptomatic, normovolemic patients	
Leukocyte-poor RBCs (LP-RBCs)	Increase red cell mass Prevent febrile reactions due to leukocyte antibodies in patients with severe and/or recurrent nonhemolytic febrile transfusion reactions Decreases the likelihood of alloimmunization to leukocyte or HLA antigens Decrease transmission of viral infections	
Deglycerolized RBCs (D-RBCs)	Increase red cell mass Storage of rare and autologous blood for more than 42 days Minimize allergic/febrile reactions Paroxysmal nocturnal hemoglobinuria	Cost precludes routine use in transfusion therapy
Fresh frozen plasma (FFP)	Reversal of Coumadin drugs Replace antithrombin III Thrombotic thrombocytopenic purpura	Volume expander Nutritional source of protein Source of immunoglobulins

INDICATIONS AND CONTRAINDICATIONS OF BLOOD AND BLOOD PRODUCTS (Contd...)

Blood and Blood Components	Indications for use	Contraindications for use
Cryoprecipitate (CRYO)	Replace isolated factor deficiencies Correct multiple coagulation factor deficiencies secondary to DIC, liver disease, and massive transfusion. von Willebrand's disease, hemophilia-A, Factor-XIII deficiency, and congenital/ acquired fibrinogen deficiency. Source of fibrin glue	
Factor VIII concentrate	Prevent/control bleeding in hemophilia-A patients with moderate to severe deficiency of Factor-VIII Hemophilia-A patients with low levels of Factor-VIII inhibitors	Treat von Willebrand's disease
Factor IX complex	Hemophilia-B Patients with Factor-VIII or IX inhibitors Congenital Factor-VII or X deficiency	Patients with liver disease
Coagulation Factor IX complex	Hemophilia-B	
Anti-inhibitor coagulation complex (AICC)	Hemophilia-A patients with high titer of Factor-VIII antibodies	
Desmopressin acetate (DDAVP)	Mild/moderate forms of hemophilia-A Certain types of von Willebrand's disease	

(Contd....)

INDICATIONS AND CONTRAINDICATIONS OF BLOOD AND BLOOD PRODUCTS (Contd...)

Blood and Blood Components	Indications for use	Contraindications for use
Platelets (PC)		
Random donor	Prophylaxis Dilutional thrombocytopenia Active bleeding due to thrombocy topenia or thrombocytopathy Thrombocytopenia due to septicemia/ hypersplenism in nonbleeding patient Thrombotic thrombocytopenic purpura	Autoimmune idiopathic thrombo-cytopenic purpura Drug-induced thrombocytopenia Untreated DIC
Single donor	Thrombocytopenia in alloimmunized patients	
Granulocyte concentrates (GC)	Documented granulocyte dysfunction Infections unresponsive to antibiotics	Patients with poor chance of bone marrow recovery Infections responsive to antibiotic therapy
Plasma substitutes albumin, plasma proteins	Volume expansion, colloid replacement	Correct nutritional deficiency

COAGULATION FACTORS

Factor	*Common Name*	*Minimum Hemostatic Level (IU/dL)*
I	Fibrinogen	50 mg/dL
II	Prothrombin	40
V	Proaccelerin	5-10
VII	Proconvertin	5-10
VIII	Antihemophilic factor	25-30
IX	Christmas factor	15-35
X	Smart-Prower factor	8-10
XII	Plasma thromboplastin antecedent (PTA)	10-20
XIII	Fibrin stabilizing factor	

REACTIVITY OF COMMON SYSTEM ANTIBODIES

Antibody Specificity	0 adult	A_2 Adult	A_1 Adult	B Adult	O Cord	O_1 Adult
Anti-I	++++	++++	++++	++++	$o/+^w$	$o/+^w$
Anti-i	$o/+^w$	$o/+^w$	$o/+^w$	$o/+^w$	++++	++++
Anti-IH	++++	+++	$o/+^w$	$o/1^+$	$o/+^w$	$o/+^w$
Anti-IT	+++	+++	++++	+++	++++	+ 1

PHYSICAL AND BIOLOGICAL PROPERTIES OF HUMAN IMMUNOGLOBULIN CLASSES

	IgG	IgA	IgM	IgD	IgE
H chain classes	7	a	m	d	e
H chain subclasses	4	2	3	4	
Constant domains	3	3	4	3	4
Exist as polymer	no	yes	yes	no	no
Molecular weight	150,000	160,000	900,000	180,000	190,000
Serum concentration (mg/dL)	1500	350	200	3	0.05
Carbohydrate (%)	3	8	12	13	12
Serum half-life (days)	23	6	5	2-8	1-5
Present in secretions	no	yes	no	no	no
Antibody activity	yes	yes	yes	no	yes
Complement fixation	yes	no	yes	no	no
Cross placenta	yes	no	no	no	no
Usual serologic characteristics	non-agglutinating	non-agglutinating	agglutinating	?	?

CHARACTERISTICS OF IgG SUBCLASSES

	IgG1	*IgG2*	*IgG3*	*IgG4*
Percent of total IgG	60-70	15-25	4-8	2-5
Serum half-life (days)	23	23	8	23
Complement fixation	yes	yes	yes	no
Cross placenta	yes	yes	yes	yes
Fc receptor on				
Macrophages	yes	no	yes	no
Neutrophils	yes	yes	yes	no
Gm groups present	yes	yes	yes	no

* Less efficient than IgG1 and IgG3

COMPONENTS IN THE CLASSIC PATHWAY OF COMPLEMENT ACTIVATION

Complement Component	*Cleavage fragment*	*Function*
Cl		
Clq		Complexes with antibody Fc region
Clr		Complexes with Clq and activates C4 and C2
ClsCls		
C2	C2a, C2b	C2b complexes with C4b to form C3 convertase

(Contd....)

COMPONENTS IN THE CLASSIC PATHWAYS OF COMPLEMENT ACTIVATION (Contd.......)

Complement Component	*Cleavage fragment*	*Function*
C3	C3a,C3b	C3b binds to membrane
	C3c, C3d	
C4	C4a, C4b	see C2 above
	C4c, C4d	
C5	C5a,C5b	C5b binds to membrane
C6		
C7		
C8		Attack sequence
C9		

FISHER-RACE GENES AND ANTIGENS

Genes and Antigens

Tibodies	**CDe**	**cDE**	**cde**	**cDe**	**cdE**	**Cde**	**CDE**	**CdE**
ti-C	+	—	—	—	—	—	+	+
ti-D	+	+	—	+	—	—	+	—
ti-E	—	+	—	—	+	—	+	+
ti-c	—	+	+	+	+	—	—	—
ti-e	+	—	+	+	—	+	—	—

ANTIHUMAN GLOBULIN DEFINITIONS

Reagent	Definition
Polyspecific (rabbit polyclonal)	Contains anti-IgG and anti-C3d; may contain other anticomplement and other anti-immunoglobulin antibodies
Polyspecific (rabbit/murine monoclonal blend)	Monoclonal anti-C3b and C3d
Anti-IgG	Contains anti-IgG with no anticomplement activity (not necessarily gamma chain specific)
Anti-IgG (heavy chain)	Contains only antibodies reactive against human gamma chains
Anti-C3d and anti-C3b (rabbit polyclonal)	Contains only antibodies reactive against the designated complement component(s) with no anti-immunoglobulin activity
Anti C3d (murine monoclonal)	Contains only antibodies reactive against the designated complement component, with no anti-immunoglobulin activity.
Anti-C3b-C3d (monoclonal)	Contains only antibodies reactive against the designated complement component, with no anti-immunoglobulin activity.

EIGHT KNOWN KELL HAPLOTYPES

Numeric	Antigens produced	Comment
KEL 2,4,7,11	k, Kpb, Jsb, K11	Very common in all populations
KEL 1,4,7,11	K, Kpb,Jsb, K11	Less common but more common in Caucasians than blacks
KEL 2,3,7,11	k, Kpa, Jsb, K11	Rare. More common in Caucasians than blacks
KEL 2,21,7,11	k, Kpc, Jsb, K11	Very Rare. Seen in Japanese

(Contd.....)

EIGHT KNOWN KELL HAPLOTYPES (Contd....)

Numeric	Antigens produced	Comment
KEl 2,3,6,11	k,Kpb,Jsa,K11	Rare. More common in blacks than Caucasians
KEL 2,4,7,10,11	k, Kpb,Jsb,Ula,K11	Very rare. Found in Finns
KEL 2,4,7,17	k, Kpb, Jsb, K17	Very rare
Ko	None	Very rare

SEROLOGIC CHARACTERISTICS OF DIFFERENT SUBGROUPS OF A

	Reactions with						
Subgroup	Human Anti-A	Anit-A, B	Anti-A1+	Anti-H	Monoclonal Anti-A	Substances(s) in Saliva if secretor	Anti-A1 in Serum
A_1	++++	++++	++++	+	++++	A and H	No
A_2	++++	++++	0	+++	++++	A and H	4%
A_{int}	++++	++++	++	+++	++++	A and H	No
A_3	++ mixed field	++ mixed field	0	++++	+++++	A and H	Few
A_x	$0/+^w$	+/++	0	++++	+++	H	Usually
A_m	$+^w$	$+^w$	0	++++	NT	A and H	No
A_{end}	$+^w$	$+^w$	0	+++++	NT	H	No
A_{el}	0	0	0	+++++	O^w	H	Few
A_{bantu}	$+^w$	$+^w$	0	++++	++	H	Usually
A_{finn}	$+^w$	$+^w$	0	++++	NT	H	All

FREQUENCIES OF THE EIGHT COMMON RH GENES

	Fishere-Race Terminology		Frequency in US Population			
Haplotype	Gene Combination	Antigenic Specificities	Whites	Blacks	Native Americans	Asians
R1	CDe	C, D,e	0.42	0.17	0.44	0.70
r	cde	c,e	0.37	0.26	0.11	0.03
R2	cDE	c,D,E	0.14	0.11	0.34	0.21
R0	cDe	c,D,e	0.04	0.44	0.02	0.03
r’	Cde	C,e	0.02	0.02	0.02	0.02
r”	cdE	c,E	0.01	0.00	0.06	0.00
RZ	CDE	C,D,E	0.00	0.00	0.00	0.06 0.01
Ry	CdE	C,E	0.00	0.00	0.00	0.00 0.00

CLASSIFICATIONS FOR D-POSITIVE RED CELLS IN INDIVIDUALS WHO PRODUCE ALLOANTI-D ANTI-D FROM D+ PEOPLE

		III			IV			V			VI						
CELLS	*II*	*a*	*b*	*c*	*a*	*a*	*b*	*a*	*b*	*c*	*i*	*ii*	*VII*	*G*	*Anti-Goa*	*Dw*	*TAR*
II	—	+	+	+	+	+	W	+	+	W	+	+	nt	+	—	—	—
IIIa	+	—	+	—	+	*	*	+	+	+	+	+	W	+	—	—	—
b	+	—	—	—	+	+	+	W	+	+	+	+	nt	—	—	—	—
c	+	—	+	—	+	+	+	+	+	+	+	+	+	+	—	—	—
IVa	—	W	+	—	—	—	—	+	+	—	+	+	+	+	+	—	—
b	—	W	+	W	—	—	—	—	+	W	+	—	nt	+	—	—	—
Va	+	—	+	—	+	W	+	—	W	—	+	—	—	+	—	+	—
c	—	—	+	—	W	—	W	—	—	—	+	—	nt	+	—	—	—
VI	—	—	+	—	+	—	+	—	—	—	—	—	—	+	—	—	—
VII	+	±	+	±	+	+	+	±	+	+	+	+	—	+	—	—	+

KELL BLOOD GROUP SYSTEM ANTIGENS

Relative Numeric	Alphabetic	Incidence	Comments
KEL1	K	Low	Antithetical to KEL2
KEL2	k	High	Antithetical to KEL1
KEL3	Kpa	Low	Antithetical to KEL4 and KEL21
KEL4	Kpb	High	Antithetical to KEL3 and KEL21
KEL5	Ku	High	Absent only from KO cells
KEL6	Jsa	Low	Antithetical to KEL7
KEL7	Jsb	High	Antithetical to KEL6
KEL10	Ula	Low	
KEL11	Cote	High	Antithetical to KEL17
KEL12	Boc	High	Para-KEL
KEL13	K13	High	Para-KEL
KEL14	San	High	Para-KEL
KEL16	"k-like"	High	
KEL17	Wka	Low	Antithetical to KEL11
KEL18	K18	High	Para-KEL
KEL19	Sub	High	Para-KEL
KEL20	Km	High	Absent only from K0 and McLeod
KEL21	Kpc	Low	Antithetical to KEL3 and KEL4
KEL22	K22	High	Para-KEL
KEL23	K23	Low	Para-KEL
KEL24	Cls	Low	Para-KEL

KEL8 (Kw), KEL9 (KL), and KEL15 (Kx) are obsolete.

BIOCHEMICAL CHARACTERISTICS OF STORED BLOOD

		CPDA-1				
	Whole Blood	Whole Blood	Red Blood Cells	AS-1	AS-3	AS-5
Days of storage	21	35	35	42	42	42
Percent viable cells (24 hours after tranasfusion)	80.0	79.0	71.0	76 (64-85)	83(±10)	78
Glucose (mmol/L)	—	—	—	31	28	—
pH (measured at 37°C)	6.84	6.98	6.71	6.6	6.5	6.8
ATP (% of initial value)	86.0	56.0 (±12)	64	58	55	
2,3-DPG (% of initial value)	44.0	<10.0	<10.0	<5.0	<10	<5
Plasma K+ (mmol/L)	21.0	27.3	78.5	6.5	NA	NA
Plasma hemoglobin (mg/L)	191	461	6580	—	—	—
Percent hemolysis	—	—	—	0.5	0.8	0.5

ORIGINAL SOLVED MCQ'S

MCQ's FOR TRANSFUSION MEDICINE

1. **Clinical assessment is not needed if blood loss is less than :**
   A. 500 ml B. 700 ml
   C. 800 ml D. 1000 ml
2. **In hemophilia, transfusion of factor __ is needed.**
   A. VI B. VII
   C. VIII D. IX
3. **Following are usually unsuitable donors, except :**
   A. Elderly B. Overweight
   C. On antibiotics D. Diabetic
4. **The blood usually donated is ———ml.**
   A. 350 B. 400
   C. 450 D. 500
5. **Which component of blood is most often separated and used and rest is retransfused.**
   A. RBC's B. WBC's
   C. Platelets D. Plasma
6. **If following test is positive in collected blood, the blood is nor transfused :**
   A. HBsAg or Anti HBs
   B. Antibodies against HIV
   C. Anti HCV
   D. None of the above
7. **Donor blood is not used if following test is positive, except :**
   A. Anti HTLV-I-II
   B. Elevated aminotransferase
   C. Rapid plasma reagent (RPR)
   D. Anti A, B antibodies

Ans. **1. A** **2. C** **3. C** **4. C** **5. C** **6. A** **7. D**

8. **Following is true about naturally occurring antibodies except :**
   A. They are usually IgM
   B. The most important are anti-A, and anti-B.
   C. React optimally at cold temperature (4°C) called cold antibodies
   D. Non reactive at 37°C
9. **The important antibodies develop in response to transfusion or by transplantal passage during pregnancy are :**
   A. IgG B. IgM
   C. IgD D. IgA
10. **The most important immune antibody is the Rh antibody i.e. anti— :**
   A. A B. B
   C. AB D. D
11. **Naturally occurring antibodies to appropriate ABO antigens are found in following, except :**
   A. HIV positive B. On immune suppressive drugs
   C. Neonates D. Pregnant
12. **The concept of universal donor is potentially dangerous as a proportion of donors (particularly of group O) possess following, except :**
   A. Immune IgG anti-A
   B. Immune IgG anti-B
   C. High titres of naturally occurring antibodies
   D. None of the above
13. **Hemolytic transfusion reaction can occur with following system except :**
   A. Lewis B. B.P
   C. I D. Lutheran
14. **The frequency of antibodies are rare with following, antigen :**
   A. Kh B. LeaLeb
   C. P1PPh D. Ii
15. **Blood grouping can be done from following except :**
   A. Saliva B. Semen
   C. Sweat D. None of the above
16. **A, B and H antigens are :**
   A. Amporphous proteins B. Lipoproteins
   C. Glycoproteins D. Glycosphingelipids

Ans. **8. D** **9. A** **10. D** **11. C** **12. D** **13. C** **14. D** **15. D** **16. C**

17. **Antigens are present in secretions (saliva, gastric juice and sweat) of about ———————% of all persons.**
A. 40 B. 60
C. 75 D. 90

18. **Which of the following group is non-secretor :**
A. SeSe B. Sese
C seSe D. se se

19. **Which is the commonest blood group in India :**
A. A B. B
C. O D. AB

20. **Which of the least common blood group :**
A. A B. B
C. O D. AB

21. **Hemolytic disease of newborn is seen with following :**
A. Kell B. Lewis
C. Lutheran D. I

22. **Hemolytic disease of new born is seen with :**
A. MNS B. Kid
C. Duffy D. All of the above

23. **Following contains both anti-A and anti-B antibodies :**
A. A B. B
C. AB D. O

24. **The proportion of A1 and A2 of group is :**
A. 90 :10 B. 80 : 20
C. 70 : 30 D. 60 : 40

25. **Anti-A and anti-B isoantibodies appear in the serum of infants by about the age of ———— months and persist thereafter.**
A. 1 B. 2
C. 3 D. 6

26. **The extract of plant ulex europaeus has potent anti———— agglutinin.**
A. A_1, B. A_2
C. B D. H

27. **The extract of plant Dolichos fiflorus has potent anti———— agglutinin.**
A. A_1 B. A_2
C. B. D. A_2B

Ans.	17. C	18. D	19. C	20. D	21. A	22. D
	23. D	24.B	25. D	26. D	27. A	

28. In acute hemolytic transfusion, the component of antibody which activates complement and causes red cell lysis is :

A. IgG B. IgM
C. IgA D. IgE

29. ABO hemolytic disease occur due to maternal anti-A and anti-B antibodies of ———isotype crossing the placenta.

A. IgG B. IgM
C. IgA D. IgD

30. The colour code used for blood group 'O' is :

A. Pink B. White
C. Yellow D. Blue

31. Autologous transfusion is accepted not less than——hours before surgery.

A. 12 B. 24
C. 48 D. 72

32. Acceptable blood in autologous donation is atleast ———% of haematocut or higher :

A. 26 B. 33
C. 46 D. 59

33. Amount to be withdrawn from a donor is calculated as donor weight (mKg) :

A. Divided by 40 multiplied by 350
B. Divided by 50 multiplied by 450
C. Divided by 70 multiplied by 550
D. Divided by 70 multiplied by 600

34. Blood donation is deferred by 2 weeks if patient has been vaccinated for following except :

A. Mumps B. Influenza
C. Measles D. Yellow fever

35. A patient who has been vaccinated for rubella, vaccination is deferred :

A. For two weeks B. For four weeks
C. For twelve months D. Not at all

36. The frequency of whole blood donation is in every ———days under normal circumstances

A. 45 B. 56
C. 65 D. 90

Ans. **28. B** **29. A** **30. D** **31. D** **32.B** **33. B**
34. B **35. B** **36. B**

37. **After platelet donation, at least ——— hours must pass before donor can give whole blood.**

A. 24 B. 48
C. 72 D. 120

38. **After plasma donation, at least——— hours must pass before donor can give whole blood.**

A. 12 B. 24
C. 48 D. 96

39. **Plasma lost during donation return to normal levels within :**

A. 24 hours B. 72 hours
C. 96 hours D. 30 days

40. **Type of donors which are maximum are :**

A. Professional B. Voluntary
C. Involuntary D. Replacement

41. **The service set up of blood bank which deals with usuing of blood to a deserving and needy recipient is :**

A. Credit B. Debit
C. A or B D. None

42. **The volume of blood which is withdrawn at a time from donor is :**

A. 200 c.c. B. 300 c.c.
C. 500 c.c. D. 540 c.c.

43. **Volume depletion in donation is replenished in :**

A. 12-24 hours B. 24-48 hours
C. 48-72 hours D. One week

44. **Hemoglobin level is replenished after donating one unit of blood in :**

A. 1-2 weeks B. 2-3 weeks
C. 3-4 weeks D. 6-8 weeks

45. **WHO norm is ——— units of blood per hospital bed.**

A. 2 B. 4
C. 5 D. 7

46. **A notification issued under Drugs and Cosmetic Act making a sample of every blood unit tested was in :**

A. 1983 B. 1985
C. 1989 D. 1991

47. **Design of blood bank should be such that the following 3 rams should be accessible to persons from outside the blood bank, except :**

A. Reception room B. Donation room
C. Refreshment room D. Rest room

Ans. **37. B** **38. C** **39. A** **40. D** **41. A** **42. B**
43. C **44. C** **45. D** **46. C** **47. C**

48. Donors should preferably be in the age group of :

A. 12-65 years B. 18-60 years
C. 18-55 years D. 12-60 years

49. In a donor, Hemoglobin (gm/dl) and PCV (%) should not be less than _________ respectively.

A. 13, 40 B. 12.5, 38
C. 12, 35 D. 12, 30

50. Donors weighing 55 kg can give about ________ ml blood.

A. 300 B. 350
C. 400 D. 450

51. For donating blood, oral temperature shall not exceed ________°C.

A. 38 B. 37.5
C. 37 D. 36.5

52. The usual interval between donation of unit of blood shall be at least ________ weeks.

A. 4 B. 6
C. 8 D. 12

53. After plasmapheresis or cytapheresis, at least ______ hours must elapse before whole blood donation.

A. 12 B. 24
C. 36 D. 48

54. Prospective donor is not accepted if patient is pregnant and lactating till _______ months :

A. 3 B. 4
C. 6 D. 9

55. Persons recently immunized with following vaccines are accepted as donor, except :

A. Toxoids B. Killed virus vaccine
C. Rickettsial vaccine D. None of the above

56. Following inoculation with attenuated virus vaccines such as polio (live) measles etc, donors are deferred for _______ weeks.

A. 1 B. 2
C. 6 D. 12

57. After a major operation, donors are not accepted until ____ months.

A. 2 B. 3
C. 6 D. 12

Ans. **48. B** **49. B** **50. D** **51. B** **52. D** **53. D**
54. C **55. D** **56. B** **57. C**

58. After a minor operation, donors are not accepted until ____ months :

A. 1. B. 2

C. 3 D. 4

59. A donor may be accepted if his/her blood transfusion causes hepatitis in a patient within 6 months and there are no other sources of infection:

A. After 12 months B. After 24 months

C. After immunoglobulin D. Never

60. A donor who has received blood or blood components during preceding __________ months shall be deferred.

A. 1 B. 2

C. 3 D. 6

61. A donor who had malaria and treated will be accepted after __________ months.

A. 2 B. 3

C. 4 D. 6

62. Following donors are revised to refrain from donation, except :

A. Tetanus B. Homosexual

C. Intravenous drug abuser D. Hepatitis B

63. Donors receiving following medicines may be accepted, except :

A. Oral contraceptives B. Beta blockers

C. Salicylates D. Antibiotics

64. On storage, the visibility of red cells from G-6-P-D deficient patient is:

A. Less B. Normal

C. Higher D. Any of the above

65. A donor with polycythemia vera is :

A. Accepted if haematocut is below 45%

B. Accepted of on medication

C. Accepted of Hb is 12 gm%

D. Never accepted

66. Acid Dextrose solution required for 300 ml blood is _____ ml :

A. 15 B. 30

C. 45 D. 60

67. The solution of Citrate-Phosphate-Dextrose required for 100 ml of blood is _________ ml.

A. 10 B. 12

C. 14 D. 18

Ans. 58. C 59. D 60. D 61. B 62. A 63. D 64. A 65. D 66. C 67. C

68. The solution of Citrate-Phosphate-Dextrose-Adenine (CPDA-I) required for 300 ml of blood is :

A. 30 B. 36
C. 42 D. 48

69. Immediately after collection, the blood shall be placed at _______ °C.

A. 2-6 B. 4-10
C. 10-12 D. 4 to 0

70. If donated blood is used as a source of platelets it should be stored at ----------------°C until platelets are separated but not more than 6 hours.

A. 12-16 B. 16-20
C. 20-24 D. 28-32

71. If the seal is broken during processing including pooling, components stored between 1-6°C must be transfused within_________hours.

A. 6 B. 12
C. 24 D. 36

72. If components of blood are stored between 20-24°C, then blood must transfused as early as possible but not beyond _____hours.

A. 6 B. 12
C. 18 D. 24

73. Cryprotective agent in most common use is :

A. Normal saline B. Na fluoride
C. Glycerol D. Mannitol

74. The method of preparation, storage, thawing and washing will ensure a viability of at least ________% of transfused cells 24 hours after transfusion.

A. 60 B. 70
C. 80 D. 90

75. Red cells can be stored frozen continuously at low temperature of ________ °C in the presence of a cryoprotective agent :

A. 1 to -4 B. -5 to -10
C. -30 to 40 D. -70 to -160

76. Platelets stored at room temperature (20-24°C) shall be suspended in approx. _______ ml of plasma.

A. 20 B. 30
C. 50 D. 100

Ans. 68. C 69. A 70. C 71. C 72. A 73. C
74. B 75. D 76. D

77. **The pH of _________or higher should be maintained throughout the storage period for ______platelets.**

A. 5.5 B. 6.0

C. 6.6 D. 7.0

78. **Platelet concentrate prepared from blood (450 ml) shall contain a minimum of ______platelets in atleast 75% of units tested on storage.**

A. 5.0×10^{10} B. 5.5×10^{10}

C. 6.0×10^{9} D. 6.5×10^{9}

79. **Granulocyte concentrate prepared by cryophoresis shall contain ______ granulocytes ($\times 10^{10}$) in 75% of units tested :**

A. 1 B. 2

C. 4.5 D. 5.0

80. **Plasma shall be separated from the whole blood at anytime upto _____ days after expiry of the whole blood.**

A. 3 B. 5

C. 7 D. 10

81. **Fresh plasma shall be separated from the whole blood and frozen solid at -40°C to -80% as early as possible and not later than _____ hours of collection.**

A. 2 B. 6

C. 12 D. 20

82. **The fresh frozen plasma shall be thawed in _______°C circulating water both or in _______°C cold room.**

A. 4 B. 10

C. 14 D. 18

83. **The cryoprecipitate cold insoluble material shall be frozen within _____ hours.**

A. 4 B. 10

C. 14 D. 18

84. **Following techniques are used to detect serologically HLA A, B and C antigens, except :**

A. Micro-lymphocytotoxicity test

B. Platelet complement fixation test

C. Leucocyte microagglutination test

D. ELISA

Ans. **77. B** **78. B** **79. A** **80. B** **81. B** **82. A**
83. A **84. D**

85. In microlymphocytotoxicity test following are isolated from peripheral blood except :

A. RBC's B. Leucocytes
C. Lymphocyte D. Platelets

86. The final lymphocyte preparation should consist of atleast _____% viable and pure lymphocytes.

A. 70 B. 80
C. 90 D. 95

87. If there is 11-30% increase in cell death over negative control %, the interpretation of the result will be :

A. Negative B. Weak negative
C. Weak positive D. Positive

88. Koa, Kob and DUZO are ______ specific antigens.

A. Lymphocytes B. Neutrophil
C. Platelet D. Red cell

89. HGA-A, HGA-2, HGA-3 are antigens, neutrophils share with :

A. Lymphocytes B. Basophils
C. Eosinophils D. Monocytes

90 Excess of EDTA affects :

A. RBC's B. Leukocytes
C. Both of the above D. None of the above

91. EDTA in excess of 2 mg/ml in blood may result in :

A. ↑PCV B. ↓MCHC
C. ↓PCV D. None of the above

92. Dipotassium salt has solubility of _____ g/L :

A. 108 B. 452
C. 914 D. 1650

93. Disodium salt has solubility of _____ g/L :

A. 78 B. 108
C. 914 D. 1726

94. The colour code used for group 'B' is ______ :

A. Blue B. Green
C. Yellow D. Pink

95. All Rh(D) negative shall be printed :

A. Blue B. Green
C. Red D. White

Ans. **85. A** **86. C** **87. B** **88. C** **89. D** **90. C**
91. C **92. D** **93. B** **94. D** **95. C**

96. **Not more than _______ numeric or alphanumeric identification shall be on a blood or component contained :**

A. 1 B. 2
C. 3 D. 4

97. **Blood group AB is given colour code of :**

A. Yellow B. Purple
C. Blue D. White

98. **In AB group patients of AB group blood is not available, group ______ preferable to _____ group as anti____ is weaker than anti______.**

A. A,B,A,B B. A,B,B,A
C. B,A,B,A D. B,A,A,B

99. **Donated blood is screened for following infections, except :**

A. HIV B. HBs Ag
C. Hepatitis C D. Malaria

100. **A typical antibodies active at _______°C of other systems are serologically signified.**

A. 37 B. 36.4
C. 35 D. 32.6

101. **Universal recipient is :**

A. 'O' negative B. 'O' positive
C. 'AB' positive D. 'AB' negative

102. **Universal donor is :**

A. 'O' negative B. 'O' positve
C. 'AB' positive D. 'AB' negative

103. **In a patient with blood group A1 with anti HI (O) the alternative blood group of first choice is :**

A. A B. B
C. O D. None of the above

104. **A patient with blood group A, B with anti-HI (O), the alternative blood group of first choice is :**

A. A1 B. B
C. A1 or B D. O

105. **A patient with blood group Rh (D) negative is in critical need of blood and Rh(D) negative blood is not available. He may be given :**

A. Rh (D) positive blood provided blood does not have anti Rh (D) antibodies.

B. Rh (D) positive blood irrespective of antibodies.

C. Rh (D) negative with anti-Rh (D) antibodies.

D. None is true.

Ans. **96. B** **97. D** **98. A** **99. D** **100. A** **101. D**
102. B **103. D** **104. C** **105. A**

106. If patient is known to have irregular antibody test the best source of blood to be transfused is :

A. From sibling
B. From his children
C. From his parents
D. Autologous

107. Blood to be transfused in hemolytic disease of newborn should not be ______ days old.

A. 1
B. 3
C. 5
D. 7

108. If exchange transfusion is required in hemolytic disease of newborn, blood should be of :

A. Same ABO and Rh type
B. Same ABO but of any Rh type
C. Any ABO but of same Rh type
D. O group and same Rh type

109. Blood transfused in hemolytic disease of newborn should be fresh to avoid :

A. Hemolysis
B. Antibodies
C. Hyperkalemia
D. Hyper masnesemia

110. In ABO Hemolytic disease of newborn, which type of blood is used :

A. 'O' group of same Rh type
B. Same ABO group of any Rh type
C. Same ABO group and Rh positive
D. Same ABO group and Rh negative

111. If baby's blood group is a A and mother's blood group is B, then blood selected for exchange transfusion is :

A. A
B. B
C. A or B
D. O

112. If baby's blood group is A and mother's blood group is AB, then blood used for exchange transfusion is :

A. A
B. A or O
C. B or O
D. O only

113. If baby's blood group is B and mother's blood group is A, then blood selected for exchange transfusion is :

A. B
B. B
C. A or B
D. O

114. If baby's blood group is AB and mother's blood group is A, then blood used for exchange transfusion is :

A. A
B. B
C. A or O
D. B or O

Ans. 106. D 107. C 108. A 109. C 110. A 111. D 112. B 113. D 114. C

115. If baby's blood group is AB and mother's blood group is O, then blood used for exchange transfusion is :

A. A B. AB
C. B D. O

116. If baby's blood group is 'O' and mother's blood group is AB, then blood to be used for exchange transfusion is :

A. A B. B
C. O D. AB

117. Blood used for patient suffering from coagulation disorder should be mainly stored upto _____ hours.

A. 24 B. 48
C. 72 D. 96

118. Old stored blood is used for neonatal exchange transfusion must not be _____ days old.

A. 1 B. 2
C. 3 D. 7

119. Blood used for massive transfusion in open heart surgery should not be _____ days old.

A. 1 B. 2
C. 3 D. 7

120. Aphaeresis is the collection of anti-coagulated whole blood from a :

A. Donor B. Patient
C. Sibling D. Donor or patient

121. Plasmapheresis is a procedure to harvest plasma from the whole blood and returning the cellular components to :

A. Blood bank B. Body
C. Patient D. None of the above

122. In plasmapheresis, total serum protein should not be blood ________ gm/dl.

A. 7.0 B. 6.8
C. 6.4 D. 6

123. In serial plasma pheresis programme, a minimum interval of _____ hours between 2 procedures and not more than two procedures in a _____ allowed.

A. 24, 3 days B. 48, 7 days
C. 72, 15 days D. 72, 30 days

Ans. **115. D** **116. C** **117. A** **118. B** **119. C** **120. D**
121. B **122. D** **123. B**

124. If a participant of serial plasmapheresis programme donates a unit of blood or if it is not possible to return red cells to donor he or she should be removed from the programme for ______ weeks :

A. 2 B. 4
C. 8 D. 12

125. If it is important to give red cells minimally, affected by physiochemical changes during storage, blood should not be older than _____ days.

A. 2 B. 3
C. 4 D. 7

126. Instead of plasma ______ is used as replacement fluid.

A. 0-9% NaCl B. 1.0% KCl
C. 7% NaHCO3 D. Na dextrose

127. During serial plasmapheresis, red blood cell loss including that of testing should not exceed _____ ml/weak.

A. 5 B. 10
C. 25 D. 50

128. Volume of plasma obtained excluding anticoagulants from a donor weighing 55 Kg should be ______ ml during on procedure of 1000 ml in a week and 25 litres in a year :

A. 250 B. 350
C. 400 D. 500

129. The procedure of separation of individual cellular components of blood is called :

A. Apheresis B. Haemopheresis
C. Plasmapheresis D. Cytapheresis

130. Platelet pheresis is deferred if platelet count is below ____ cumm :

A. 150000 B. 180000
C. 200000 D. 220000

131. Persons who have ingested aspirin within ______ hours are not suitable for platelet pheresis :

A. 24 B. 48
C. 72 D. 96

132. Granulocyte counts should be at least_____ Cumm for satisfactory yield for leukapheresis :

A. 3000 B. 4000
C. 45000 D. 5000

Ans. **124. C** **125. C** **126. A** **127. C** **128. D** **129. A**
130. A **131. A** **1 2. B**

133. **Extra corporeal blood volume should not exceed _____% of the donor's estimated blood volume.**

A. 10 B. 12

C. 15 D. 20

134. **Interval between two cytapheresis shall be _____ hours.**

A. 24 B. 48

C. 72 D. 96

135. **Not more than _____ ml of plasma should be removed per 7 days.**

A. 500 B. 750

C. 1000 D. 1250

136. **Red blood cell loss incidental to the procedure shall not be more than _____ ml per week.**

A. 10 B 25

C. 50 D. 75

137. **Whole blood, red cell concentrate shall be transported in a manner that will maintain a temperature of _______°C ± 2°C.**

A. 4 B. 10

C. 14 D. 18

138. **Platelet/granulocyte concentrate stored at 20-24°C should be transported at about _____ °C.**

A. 4-8 B. 10-14

C. 20-24 D. 28-32

139. **Whole blood shall be stored at _____°C in bottles or bags.**

A. 2-4 B. 8-10

C. 14-16 D. 18-20

140. **Whole blood collected in anticoagulant citrate-phosphate-dextrose solution shall have an expiry date, not exceeding______days after phlebotomy :**

A. 14 B. 21

C. 30 D. 45

141. **Whole blood collected in anticoagulant citrate-phosphate-dextrose with adenine (CPDA-I) shall have an expiry date not exceeding _____ days after phlebotomy :**

A. 21 B. 35

C. 45 D. 60

142. **Whole blood in heparin solution shall have an expiry period not exceeding _____ days after collection.**

A. 1 B. 2

C. 3 D. 4

Ans. **133. C** **134. B** **135. C** **136. B** **137. B** **138. C**
139. A **140. B** **141. B** **142. B**

143. Red cell concentrate shall be stored at _____°C.

A. 2-4 B. 8-10
C. 14-16 D. 18-20

144. The expiry date for glycerolized frozen red cells is _______.

A. 3 months B. 6 months
C. 1 year D. 3 years

145. Frozed red cells as stored at temperature lower than _____°C.

A. -150 B. -70
C. -4 D. 4

146. Leukocyte poor red cells should be stored at _______°C.

A. 2-6 B. 6-10
C. 10-14 D. 14-18

147. The storage temperature of granulocyte is 20-24°C which is ______ that of platelet concentrate.

A. Higher than B. Lower than
C. Same as D. Any of the above

148. Single donor plasma shall be stored as liquid plasma at 2-6°C for no more than _____ days.

A. 2 B. 3
C. 5 D. 10

149. The components shall be stored at -40°C or below and shall be stored no longer than _____ months.

A. 6 B. 9
C. 12 D. 18

150. The recipient's and donor's blood samples must be kept for ____ days at 2°C to 6°C after each transfusion.

A. 3 B. 5
C. 7 D. 14

151. Blood must not be allowed to warm above ______°C during storage or transportation.

A. 6 B. 10
C. 14 D. 36

152. Blood should not be allowed to cool below _______°C during storage or transportation.

A. 0 B. 2
C. 6 D. 10

Ans. **143. A** **144. D** **145. B** **146. A** **147. C** **148. C**
149. C **150. C** **151. B** **152. B**

153. **All units for reissue must be kept at 4-6°C for _____ hours for observation.**
A. 12 B. 24
C. 36 D. 48

154. **Single donor fresh frozen plasma is thawed at temperature between :**
A. 30-37°C B. 24-28°C
C. 18-24°C D. 2-6°C

155. **Rh (D) negative woman should receive Rh immune globulin preferably within _____ hours following amniocentesis :**
A. 6 B. 12
C. 24 D. 72

156. **Massive transfusion is defined as the replacement of atleast _____ blood volume with blood components within 24 hours period :**
A. One third B. Half
C. One D. Two

157. **Citrate toxicity causes cardiac dysfunction due to :**
A. Hyponatremia B. Hyperkalemia
C. Hypocalcemia D. Hyperphosphatemia

158. **A normothermic adult with a normally functioning liver can tolerate 1 unit of whole blood every _____ minute without needing supplemental calcium.**
A. 1 B. 2
C. 3 D. 5

159. **Calcium may be warranted to be added if there is following, except :**
A. Hypothermia B. Severe liver disease
C. Acute heart failure D. Acute renal failure

160. **Calcium supplement is gives in the form of following, except :**
A. Gluconate B. Chloride
C. Oxalate D. None of the above

161. **Citrate toxicity causes cardiac dysfunction due to :**
A. Hyponatremia B. Hyperkalemia
C. Hypocalcemia D. Hyperphosphatemia

162. **A normothermic adult with a normally functioning liver can tolerate 1 unit of whole blood every _____ minute without needing supplemental calcium.**
A. 1 B. 2
C. 3 D. 5

Ans. **153. B** **154. A** **155. D** **156. C** **157. C** **158. D**
159. D **160. C** **161. C** **162. D**

163. Calcium may be warranted to be added if there is following except :

A. Hypothermia B. Severe liver disease

C. Acute heart failure D. Acute renal failure

164. Calcium supplement is gives in the form of following, except :

A. Gluconate B. Chloride

C. Oxalate D. None of the above

165. Massive transfusion may result in :

A. Metabolic alkalosis B. Metabolic acidosis

C. Respiratory alkalosis D. Respiratory acidosis

166. Neonates undergoing exchange transfusion routinely requires fresh blood i.e. blood less than _______ old otherwise hyperkalemia may result.

A. 7 days B. 14 days

C. 20 days D. 1 month

167. 0.5-1.0% solution of hypochloride dissolved in 0.5% anionic or non-ionic detergent is the best for general purpose disinfectant if contact is maintained for atleast ______ min :

A. 5 B. 10

C. 15 D. 30

168. Best way for disposal of blood and lab material is :

A. Chemical B. Autoclaving

C. Boiting D. Incineration

169. DP, DQ, and DR refers to class ______ of HLA.

A. I B. II

C. III D. IV

170. Platelets contains class______ of HLA :

A. I B. II

C. III D. IV

171. Alpha chain of polyheptide in HLA class II weight of ______ deltons :

A. 29000 B. 34000

C. 37000 D. 45000

172. Beta chain has a molecular weight of _______ deltons.

A. 23000 B. 27000

C. 29000 D. 32000

173. HLA Class I interacts with ______ lymphocytes.

A. CD4 B. CD6

C. CD8 D. CD10

Ans. 163. D 164. C 165. B 166. A 167. D 168. B
169. B 170. A 171. B 172. C 173. C

174. **HLA Class-II interacts with ______ lymphocytes :**
A. CD4 B. CD6
C. CD8 D. CD10

175. **MHA is also known as HLA complex and is equivalent to the murine _____ complex.**
A. H-1 B. H-2
C. H-3 D. H-4

176. **C2, C4 and Bf are complement system of class______ proteins.**
A. I B. II
C. III D. IV

177. **Beta-2 microglobulin is coded on chromosome______ :**
A. 13 B. 15
C. 17 D. 19

178. **Which of the following HLA has maximum number of specificities :**
A. A B. B
C. D D. DR

179. **Typical class-I gene is encoded by ______ exams.**
A. 6 B. 7
C. 8 D. 9

180. **The alpha and beta chains of the Class-II molecules encoded within _____ kil doses of the MHC complex.**
A. 1000 B. 1100
C. 1200 D. 1300

181. **A typical alpha gene of class II protein contains :**
A. 3 B. 4
C. 5 D. 7

182. **To determine ESR, sodium citrate is used in one volume with _____ volumes of venous blood.**
A. 2 B. 3
C. 4 D. 6

183. **Irrespective of anticoagulant, films made from than _______ min at room temperature (18-25°C) :**
A. 30 B. 45
C. 60 D. 90

184. **The red cells are little affected by standing upto ______ hour at room temperature (18°-25°C).**
A. 1 B. 3
C. 6 D. 12

Ans. **174. A** **175. B** **176. C** **177. B** **178. B** **179. C**
180. B **181. C** **182. C** **183. C** **184. C**

185. Gross lipemia may result in positive error of upto _____ g/L of Hemoglobin estimation.

A. 1 B. 2
C. 3 D. None of the above

186. Normal range of hemoglobin is maximum in :

A. Preterm infant B. Full term infant
C. Children 3-6 years D. Elderly above 70 years

187. Total red cound is maximum in :

A. Men B. Women
C. Full term infant D. Children at 3 months of age

188. MCV may be higher in following, except :

A. Normal newborn B. Down's syndrome
C. Hyperthyroidism D. Folate deficiency

189. MCV is highest at :

A. Birth B. 3 months of age
C. 6 years of age D. 65 years and above

190. TLC is maximum in :

A. Newborn B. 3 months of age
C. 12 months of age D. 60 years of age

191. Dunger's solution is used to estimate :

A. PCV B. ESR
C. Absolute Eosinophil count D. MCHC

192. Leukopenia may be seen in following, except :

A. Cirrhosis of liver B. Rheumatoid arthritis
C. Uremia D. Scrub typhus

193. Epsilon-4 is _______ hemoglobin.

A. HbF B. Adult
C. Gower-I D. Gower-II

194. Howell Jolly bodies may occasionally be seen in :

A. Thalassemia major B. Thalassemia intermedia
C. Thalassemia minor D. Iron deficiency anemia

195. Hemosiderin may be absent in :

A. Iron deficiency anemia
B. Thalassemia major
C. Thalassemia intermedia
D. Thalassemia minor

Ans. 185. C 186. B 187. A 188. C 189. A 190. A
191. C 192. C 193. C 194. A 195. A

196. **Half life of tissue factor is ____ hours.**
A. 48-72 B. 90-120
C. 10-12 D. 14-16

197. **Half life of AHF is about _____ hours.**
A. 2-6 B. 6-10
C. 10-12 D. 14-16

198. **Which of the following coagulation factor has shortest half life :**
A. I B. V
C. VII D. IX

199. **Fletcher factor is :**
A. Proconvertin B. Hageman factor
C. Prekallikrein D. Thromboplastin precursor

200. **Following factors have serino protease as active form, except :**
A. I B. II
C. IX D. XII

201. **Which of the following factor acts on intrinsic, extrinsic and common pathways :**
A. Christmas factor B. Stuart-Proner factor
C. Fletcher factor D. Fitzgerals factor

202. **Fitzgerals factor (HMWK), a cofactor has a half life of _____ hours.**
A. 2-8 B. 12-24
C. 48-52 D. 90-110

203. **Macrophages synthesize the following factors, except :**
A. VII B. IX
C. X D. XIII

204. **Following factors require vit K for activation, except :**
A. VII B. VIII
C. IX D. X

205. **Megakaryocytes synthesize the following factors, except :**
A. Fibrinogen B. V
C. VII D. XIII

206. **Following factor belongs to prothrombin group :**
A. I B. II
C. V D. VIII

207. **Mature megakaryocyte has a size of ______ μm in diameter.**
A. 20-50 B. 70-110
C. 120-160 D. 160-210

Ans.	196. C	197. C	198. C	199. C	200. A	201. B
	202. C	203. D	204. B	205. C	206. B	207. A

208. Total Red Cell Volume (TRCV) in women is _____ ml/kg :

A. 28 B. 32
C. 36 D. 38

209. In renal failure, following cell may be seen :

A. Spherocyte B. Elliptocyte
C. Burr cell D. Acanthecyte

210. Pappenheimer's bodies may be seen in :

A. Oxidative hemolysis B. Sideroblastic anemia
C. Lead poisoning D. Mercury poisoning

211. In liver disease, following may be seen :

A. Howell Jolly bodies B. Acanthocyte
C. Elliptocyte D. Sickle cell

212. In RBC membrane, which has the minimum amount :

A. Carbohydrate B. Lipid
C. Protein D. All have equal percentage

213. Luebering-Rapofort shunt generates :

A. NADH B. NADPH
C. 2,3 DPG D. All of the above

214. A typical beta chain gene of class II molecule is similar to the alpha chain gene but has ______ extra exons for the cytoplasmic tail :

A. 1 B. 2
C. 3 D. 5

215. Processes of the innate immune system inside :

A. Production of antibody upon exposure to foreign antigens.
B. Delayed hypersensitivity reactions.
C. Synthesis of complement proteins.
D. Phagocytosis of viral particles.

216. The change in production of IgM to IgG is an example of :

A. Epitope switching
B. Isotype switching
C. Immune surveillance
D. Antibody specificity

217. Which of the following is an example of immunity :

A. Lymphokine production
B. Antibody production
C. Phagocytosis
D. Graft rejection

Ans. 208. B 209. C 210. B 211. B 212. A 213. C
214. A 215. D 216. B 217. C

218. The tuberculin skin test reaction is an example of what type of immune response :

A. Production of humoral antibody
B. Antibody-independent cell mediated cytotoxicity
C. Delayed hypersensitivity
D. Antibody-dependent cell mediated cyto-toxicity

219. In humans B-cells mature in :

A. The bursa
B. The liver
C. The bone marrow
D. The thymus

220. Tissue macrophages can be found in :

A. The spleen
B. The liver
C. Lymph nodes
D. All of the above

221. Human B-cells carry surface markers*:

A. Immunoglobulin
B. Fc receptors
C. CD4 antigen
D. β-antigen

222. Analysis of T-cell subsets has shown that approximately ______% of T cells are helper T-cells :

A. 35
B. 50
C. 65
D. 80

223. In general, antibody produced to T-independent antigens is :

A. IgA
B. IgD
C. IgG
D. IgM

224. In order for an immune process to take place, the antigen-processing cells and helper T cells must have compatible :

A. Fc receptors
B. Major histocompatibility antigens
C. Monokines
D. CD4 antigens

225. Which of the following is true of immunoglobulins (Ig) of the IgM class :

A. They are the most abundant in human serum.
B. They exist only as monomers.
C. They are the only Ig class that crosses the placenta.
D. Each molecule has a J chain.

226. The major factor affecting the electrostatic repulsion between red cells is the :

A. Dielectric constant
B. pH of the medium
C. Zeta potential
D. Immunoglobulin class

Ans. **218. C** **219. C** **220. D** **221. A** **222. C** **223. D**
224. B **225. C** **226. C**

227. An agglutination reaction in which there are many small agglutinates in a turbid background would be graded as :

A. 1+ B. 2+
C. 3+ D. 4+

228. The direct antiglobulin test is useful for which of the following :

A. The detection of hemolytic disease of the newborn.
B. The identification of unknown serum allo-antibodies.
C. The identification of antigens on the surface of red cells.
D. The determination of compatibility between donor and recipient red cells.

229. A patient has been transfused with two units of blood. The recipient was previously sensitized to the antigens present on the trnasfused red cells and has an anamnestic response. Which of the following would most probably by true of this case :

A. The transfused red cell will survive normally.
B. The patient will have no physical signs.
C. The patient will shift from IgM to IgG production.
D. Antibody production will not take place for at least two weeks.

230. Interleukin-3 is a substance that stimulates T-cell proliferation and is an example of :

A. A red cell alloantibody
B. A skin-reactive factor
C. A red cell membrane glycophorin
D. A lymphokine

231. The "attach sequence" of the classic complement pathway includes :

A. Clq, Clr, and Cls B. C2,C3 and C4
C. Cl through C9 D. C6 through C9

232. The following statement best describes which of the antiglobulin reagents :

Contains anti-IgG and anti-C3d; may contain other anticomplement and other anti-immunoglobulin activities

A. Polyspecific antihuman globulin
B. Anti-IgG
C. Anti-IgG (heavy chain)
D. Anti-C3d (murine monoclonal)

Ans. **227. A** **228. A** **229. C** **230. D** **231. D** **232. A**

233. NK cells arise from which precursor cell :

A. Hematopoietic stem cell

B. Granulocyte/monocyte precursor

C. B-cell progenitor

D. Lymphopoietic stem cell

234. Which of the following statement is not true of the H-antigen :

A. Inheritance of the H antigen is necessary for the normal expression of the ABO antigens.

B. The amount of H antigen varies for different ABO types

C. The antibody directed toward the H-antigen (anti-H) is naturally occurring in the serum of most adults.

D. H. antigen may be present in the secretions.

235. Which of the following is true of type-II precursor chains :

A. They have a β1—>linkage between the terminal sugars.

B. They are found only as glycolipids on the red cell membrane.

C. They are found only as glycoproteins in body secretions.

D. They are found both as glycoproteins in body secretions and as glycolipids in the red cell surface.

236. An individual has the following ABH genotype : AO, hh. Which of the following antigens would be present on the red cells of this individual:

A. A only B. A and H

C. A and O D. None of the above

237. A group- A man marries a group AB woman. The father of the group-A man was group O. What possible ABO groups would be expected from this matching :

A. A, B, AB, and O B. A and B

C. A, B and AB D. A and AB

238. Given the data in question 4 above, what percentage of the offspring could be expected to be group A :

A. 5% B. 25%

C. 50% D. 75%

239. Which of the following is true regarding the ABO serology ofnew-borns:

A. ABH antigens are complex branched structures.

B. ABH antigens are strongly expressed at 5 to 6 weeks gestation.

C. ABO antibodies are produced at birth.

D. None of the above.

Ans. **233. D** **234. C** **235. B** **236. B** **237. D** **238. B** **239. A**

240. Which of the following is true of anti-A,B but not true of anti-A and anti-B:

A. Anti A, B efficiently binds complement

B. Anti A, B is present in the serum of group O individuals.

C. Anti-A, B is clinically significant

D. Anti A, B is predominantly IgG

241. A patient has the following serologic results :

Anti-A	Anti-B	Anti-A, B	A1 cells	B cells
4+	0	4+	2+	4+

Which of the following causes would be the best explanation for these results :

A. An elderly patient

B. A subgroup of A

C. Hypogammaglobulinemia

D. Deterioration of reagents

242. A patient has the following ABO typing results :

Anti-A	Anti-B	Anti-A,B	A1 Cells	B Cells
4+	4+	4+	O	O

This patient's ABO blood type is :

A. O

B. A

C. AB

D. Can not determine with the information given

243. Given the typing results in question above, indicate what ABO type red cells (plasma removed) could be safely selected for transfusion to this patient :

A. AB B. AB or O

C. AB, O,A, or B D. O

244. The products of genes inherited at the ABO locus are :

A. Carbohydrates B. Glycolipids

C. Transferases D. Kinases

245. The immunodominant sugar that confers B-blood group specificity is :

A. L-Fucose B. D-Galactose

C. N-Acetylgalactosamine D. L-Glucose

246. The O-gene has no detectable product and is therefore termed as :

A. Recessive B. Dominant

C. Co-dominant D. Amorphic

Ans. 240. D 241. A 242. D 243. B 244. C 245. D 246. A

247. A transfusion error in which group-A blood is transfused to a group O recipient could result in :

A. Rapid destruction of transfused red cells

B. Renal failure

C. Disseminated intravascular coagulation

D. All of the above

248. In the following which is the most probable examination for these results :

A. A warm autoantibody B. Rouleaux

C. A transfusion reaction D. The Bombay phenotype

249. Which of the following tests would be the most useful in resolving the problem in question 10 above :

A. Typing with Dolichos bifforus lectin

B. Typing with Ulex europaeus lectin

C. An eluate from patient's cells

D. Prewarmed techniques

250. All of the following statements are true regarding the Lewis in blood group system, except :

A. Lewis antigens are soluble antigens found in body fluids.

B. Lewis phenotypes in the secretions result from the interaction of the secretor and Lewis genes.

C. All Lewis antigens are type-I structures.

D. Lewis phenotypes in the secretions depend upon the interaction of ABO genes and Lewis genes.

251. Which of the following statements is true of the secretor system :

A. The gene Se is necessary for the secretion of soluble Le substance.

B. Approximately 20 per cent of the population are secretors.

C. Homozygous sese individuals secrete ABH antigens.

D. Secretion of the Leb antigen subsance depends upon the interaction of the Lewis and secretor genes.

252. The Se genes code for the production of which of the following enzymes :

A. D-Glucosyltransferase

B. D-Galactosyltransferase

C. N-Acetylgalactosyltransferase

D. L-Fucosyltransferase

Ans. **247. C** **248. B** **249. A** **250. D** **251. D** **252. D**

253. Type-I H antigen in secretion is a product of which of the following genes :

A. Le B. H

C. Se D. le

254. Most newborns type as which of the following Lewis phenotypes :

A. Le (a-b) B. Le (a+b-)

C. Le (a-b+) D. Le (a+b+)

255. Which statement is true regarding anti-Led:

A. It is produced only by Le (a-b) secretors.

B. It reacts only with the red cells of Le (a-b-) secretors.

C. It is produced only by Le (a-b+) secretors.

D. It reacts only with the red cells of Le (a+ b) secretors.

Use the following answer key for questions 256 to 264 below :

A. 1 and 2 are correct

B. 1, 2 and 3 are correct

C. Only 2 is correct

D. All of the responses are correct

256. A patient has the following genotype : AO, sese, Lele, Hh. Which of the following soluble antigens is/are present in the saliva :

A. A B. Le^a

C. H D. Le^b

257. Using the information in question 7 above. Which of the antigens listed below is/are present on the red blood cells of this patient :

A. A B. Le^a

C. H D. Le^b

258. A patient has the following genotype : OO, SeSe, lele, Hh. Which of the antigens listed below would be present in the saliva :

A. Type I H B. Type II H

C. Le^a D. Le^b

259. A patient has group A Le (a-b-) red cells.
Which of the following statements is/are true regarding this patient?

A. The patient is a secretor.

B. The patient has group A substance in his or her saliva.

C. The patient has some Lea antigen in his or her saliva.

D. The patient has inherited at least one H gene.

Ans. **253. C** **254. A** **255. B** **256. C** **257. B** **258. A** **259. D**

260. Which of the following statements is/are true of anti-Lea:

A. It is made by Le (a-b) secretors.

B. It is usually clinically insignificant.

C. It sometimes activates complement.

D. It causes severe hemolytic disease of the newborn.

261. Which of the following cells would be expected to react strongly with anti-LebH :

A. A^1 Le (a - b +) B. O Le (a - b +)

C. O Le (a - b -) D. A1 Le (a + b -)

262. Which of the following statements describe anti-I :

A. It is a fairly common autoantibody.

B. It reacts optimally at 4°C

C. It is associated with cold agglutinin disease

D. It may be associated with Mycoplasma pneumoniae infection

263. Which of the following antigens is/are present on the red cells of an individual of the P_1 phenotype :

A. P_1 B. P

C. P^k D. P_2

264. Which of the following statements is/are true regarding anti-P1?

A. It is usually clinically insignificant

B. It is produced by P2 individuals

C. It shows variable reactivity with a panel of random P1 positive red cells

D. It is inhibited by hydatid cyst fluid

265. The specificity of the antibody described by Landsteiner and Wiener that was produced in rabbits injected with Rhesus monkey red cells was later found to be :

A. Anti-D B. Anti-C

C. Anti-Lw D. Anti-Rh29

266. Anti-D is a clinically significant antibody because :

A. It is capable of activating complement

B. It is naturally occurring in all D-negative healthy adults

C. It can cause hemolytic transfusion reactions

D. It does not cross the placenta

Ans. 260. B 261. C 262. D 263. A 264. D 265. C 266. C

267. A patient has the following Rh antigen typing (phenotyping) results : D+, C+, E- c-, e+. The patient could have which of the following Rh genotypes :

A. R1R1 B. R2r
C. rr D. r'r

268. The frequency of the R0 gene in the white population is :

A. 0.42 B. 0.37
C. 0.14 D. 0.04

269. The frequency of the r gene in the black population is 0.26. Given a sample of 50 persons from this population, how many would you predict to be rr:

A. 3 B. 6
C. 9 D. 12

270. High-grade Du phenotypes are often associated with :

A. The inheritance of R1 or R2 variant genes
B. The inheritance of a variant R0 gene
C. A cis-position effect
D. A transposition effect.

271. A patient types as D-negative with high-protein anti-D at immediate spin and 37°C incubation. The test is positive at the antihuman globuli phase of testing. The Rh control is negative throughout. This patient should receive :

A. D-positive blood only
B. D-negative blood only
C. Either D-positive or D-negative blood
D. No blood until further testing is performed to determine the D type of the patient

272. Saline anti-D cannot be used for Du testing because :

A. It is predominantly IgG.
B. It is predominantly IgM
C. It may contain contaminating antibodies
D. Both B and C are correct

273. The most common cause of false-positive anti-D testing is :

A. The deterioration of reagents
B. Failure to follow manufacturer's directions
C. Spontaneous agglutination of red cells due to a positive DAT
D. Rouleaux formation

Ans. 267. A 268. D 269. A 270. D 271. B 272. D 273. C

274. Which of the following Rh genotypes would be positive for the compound antigen ce(f) :

A. CDe/cDE
B. cDE/Cde
C. cde/cde
D. All of the above

275. Which of the following is true of amorph type Rh null patients :

A. Are LW (a-b-)
B. Have abnormal red cell survival
C. Demonstrate stomatocytes in peripheral blood smears
D. All of the above

276. Patient number 1 has the following genotype : Cde/CDe, LWnLWn. Patient number 2 has the following genotype : Cde/cde. LWaLWa. Which of the following statements best describes the relative expression of LW antigens by these patients :

A. Patient number 1 will produce more LWa than patient number 2.
B. Patient number 1 will produce less LWa than patient number 2.
C. Both patients will produce the same amount of LWa.
D. Neither patient will produce LWa.

277. The mode of inheritance of the Kell antigens K (KEL1) and k (KEL 2) is :

A. X-linked dominant
B. X-linked recessive
C. Autosomal recessive
D. Autosomal co-dominant

278. Which of the following Kell haplotypes has never been identified :

A. K, Kpb, Jsb, K11
B. K, Kpa, Jsb, K11
C. k, Kpb, Jsb, K11
D. k, Kpa, Jsb, K11

279. Kell system antigens are inherited as haplo types that are responsible for the production of multiple Kell system antigens. This can best be explained by which of the following statements :

A. Kpa, Jsa, and K are low-incidence antigens.
B. Kpa, Kpb, and Kpc arise from alternate genes as a single sublocus.
C. Kell loci and closely linked.
D. Some Kell haplotypes are more common in certain races than in others.

280. In vitro preparation of K0 cells can be accomplished by the treatment of red cells with which of the following :

A. Ficin
B. Dithiothreitol plus cystine-activated papain (ZZAP)
C. 2-Aminothylisothiouronium bromide (AET)
D. Both B and C are correct

Ans. 274. C 275. C 276. A 277. D 278. B 279. C 280. D

281. Which of the following is true of the antibody anti-Kx:
A. It does not react with red cells from patient with the McLeod phenotype
B. It reacts strongly with K0 red cells
C. Both A and B are correct
D. Neither A nor B is correct

282. Which of the following is associated with the MC Leod syndrome :
A. Reticulocytosis and decreased haptoglobin levels
B. Increased levels of creatinine phosphokinase (MM band)
C. Both A and B are correct
D. Neither A nor B are correct

283. Genes at the MN locus are responsible for the production of which of the following :
A. MN sialoglycoprotein
B. Glycophorin-A
C. A transmembrane, glycosylated protein
D. All of the above

284. The inheritance of two Engenes result in :
A. The absence of the Mn sialoglycoprotein on the red cells.
B. Increased expression of Mn antigens on the red cells.
C. The absence of the Ss sialoglycoprotein on the red cells.
D. The diminished expression of the U antigen on the red cells.

285. An individual of the Nsu/Msu genotype lacks which of the following antigens:
A. S
B. M
C. N
D. Ena

286. Which of the following techniques/reagents may be useful in increasing the reactivity of anti-M:
A. Papain pretreated cells
B. Anticomplement antihuman globulin reagents
C. Acidified serum techniques
D. Heterozygous MN cells

287. Of the following MNSs system antibodies, which is almost always cold-reacting, IgM, and clinically insignificant :
A. Anti-S
B. Anti-U
C. Anti-s
D. Anti-N

Ans. **281. C** **282. C** **283. D** **284. A** **285. A** **286. C** **287. D**

288. Anti-Fy3 reacts with cells from individuals with which of the following genotypes :

A. FyFy
B. Fy4Fy4
C. Both A and B
D. Neither A nor B

289. Which of the following techniques/reagents is useful in the detection of anti-Fya:

A. Heat treatment of red cells at 56°C
B. Ficin pretreatment of red cells
C. Indirect antiglobulin technique
D. Incubation at room temperature and below

290. Anti-Fy and anti-Fy are implicated in which of the following :

A. Hemolytic transfusion reactions
B. Hemolytic disease of the newborn
C. Both A and B
D. Neither A nor B

291. Which of the following genes gives rise to weakened form of the Fyb antigen:

A. Fy
B. Fya
C. Fy3
D. Fy4

292. Which of the following red cells phenotypes would be the least susceptible to infection with Plasmodium vivax :

A. Fy (a-b-)
B. Fy (a+b+)
C. Fy (a-b+)
D. Fy (a+B-)

293. Which of the following techniques/reagents would be the least useful in the detection of anti Jka:

A. Low ionic strength saline (LISS)
B. Proteolytic enzymes
C. Polyethylene glycol (PEG)
D. Saline room temperature

294. All of the following statements are true of the anti-jka except :

A. It is often implicated in delayed hemolytic transfusion reactions.
B. The strength of in vitro reactions correlates well with the degree of in vivo red cells destruction.
C. It often reacts only with homozygous Jka-positive red cells.
D. It decreases in strength during storage.

Ans. 288. D 289. C 290. C 291. B 292. A 293. D 294. B

295. The Lutheran null phenotype may be inherited by which of the following mechanisms :

A. Inheritance of a dominant suppressor gene.
B. Inheritance of two recessive null genes at the Lu locus.
C. Inheritance of a gene on the X- chromosome.
D. All of the above.

296. Which of the following is true of the Lutheran blood group system :

A. Anti-Lu is often naturally occurring.
B. Anti-Lu is associated with severe hemolytic transfusion reactions.
C. Anti-Lu and anti-Lu are frequently implicated in hemolytic disease of the newborn.
D. The Lua antigen is a high-incidence antigen.

297. Which of the following antigens is destroyed proteolytic enzymes :

A. K
B. Xg^a
C. JK^a
D. Lu

298. Which of the following is a low-incidence antigen in the white population :

A. Yta (Cartwright)
B. Coa (Colton)
C. k (KEL2 or Cellano)
D. Di (Diago)

299. All of the following statements are true regarding Chido and Rogers, except :

A. They are antigenic determinants of human complement C4.
B. Antigens are well developed on cord cells.
C. Antibodies are high-titer, low-avidity anti-bodies.
D. Antibodies can be neutralized by fresh human serum.

300. Which of the following is classified as a high-titer, low-avidity antibody:

A. Anti-Fy^a
B. Anti-L_u^b
C. Anti-D_i^a
D. Anti-C_s^a

301. How many specific gene products have been described for HLA-B27:

A. 2
B. 4
C. 5
D. 7

302. It is now known that the MHC complex is inherited on the :

A. Short arm of chromosome 6.
B. Short arm of chromosome 8.
C. Long arm of chromosome 9.
D. Long arm of chromosome 12.

Ans. **295. D** **296. A** **297. C** **298. D** **299. B** **300. D** **301. D** **302. A**

303. Class-I epitopes are composed of :

A. Two heavy chains and two light chains
B. Two heavy chains and one light chain
C. One heavy chain and two light chains
D. One heavy chain and one light chain

304. Which of the following HLA antigens corresponds to Bgb:

A. HLA-B7 B. HLA-B17
C. HLA-B27 D. HLA-A28

305. HLA-E, -F, -G, and -H are newly recognized molecules in :

A. Class-I B. Class-II
C. Class-III D. Class-IV

306. Class-II antigen expression :

A. Has a wide distribution and is found on all nucleated cells.
B. Is restricted and only red cells possess the antigens.
C. Is limited to immunologically active cells and platelets.
D. Is limited to immunologically active cells.

307. C2, C4, and factor B are inactive precursor molecules inherited in which region of the MHC complex :

A. Class-I B. Class-II
C. Class-III D. Class-IV

308. A strong linkage disequilibrium exists between :

A. HLA-A1 and HLA-B8 B. HLA-A2 and HLA-B12
C. HLA-A19 and HLA-B27 D. HLA-A1 and HLA-B12

309. Which assay is commonly used to identify serologically defined antigens :

A. MLC B. CDC
C. RFLP D. PCR

310. Which of the following is used to recover lymphocytes when performing a density gradient separation :

A. DMSO B. Ficoll-Hypaque
C. Trypan Blue D. Eosin Y

311. What is the optimal lymphocyte concentration used in CDC testing :

A. 1000 to 2000 cells per mL
B. 10,000 to 20,000 cells per mL
C. 1 to 2 x 106 cells per mL
D. 1 to 2 x 108 cells per mL

Ans. **303. D** **304. B** **305. A** **306. D** **307. C** **308. A**
309. B **310. B** **311. C**

312. A purified suspension of B-lymphocytes is reused for :

A. Class I antigen typing
B. HLA-Dr and HLA-DQ antigen typing
C. C2,C4 and Factor-B typing
D. All HLA testing procedures

313. An MLC test is used to :

A. Determine Class-I compatibility between donor and patient.
B. Determine the ability of an individual to stimulate blast production with autologous cells.
C. Determine Class-II compatibility between donor and patient.
D. Determine nucleotide sequence of Class-II alleles.

314. For solid organ transplants, recipients and donors are often tested for :

A. HLA-A, -B, and-DR antigens
B. HLA-A and -B antigens
C. HLA-DR antigens only
D. HTLA antigens

315. When a child inherits a trait that neither parents has, it is regarded as :

A. A direct exclusion
B. An indirect exclusion
C. Inconclusive
D. Unlikely

316. A disease association exists between :

A. HLA-B5 and idiopathic hemochromatosis
B. HLA-B27 and ankylosing spondylitis
C. HLA-DR2 and narcolepsy
D. HLA-DR5 and insulin-dependent diabetes mellitus

317. A potential kidney transplant recipient and his siblings are typed for HLA-A and HLA-B antigens. What are the most probable haplotypes of the potential recipient :

Patient :	AI, 3	B5,7
Sibling 1 :	A1, x	B5,8
Sibling 2 :	A3, 10	B7, 12
Sibling 3 :	A1, 10	B8, 12

A. A1, B7/A3, B5
B. A1, B5/Ax, B7
C. A1, B5/A3, B7
D. A1, A3/B5, B7

Ans. 312. B 313. C 314. A 315. A 316. B 317. C

318. Given the MLC results (listed below in counts per minute) which sibling would be the best match for the proposed renal transplant :

X	Patient	Sib 1	Sib 2	Sib 3
Patient	200	300	10,000	19,500
Sib 1	300	200	12,500	8,500
Sib 2	10,500	12,000	200	11,000
Sib 3	18,000	8,000	10,500	200

A. Sibling 1
B. Sibling 2
C. Sibling 3
D. Not enough information given

319. Based on the results below, one would conclude that :

Phenotype

Mother	A9, 11; B8, B27
Alleged father	A1, A9; B12, B35
Child	A9, A10, B12, B27

A. There are no exclusions and the alleged man is the biologic father.
B. There is a first-order exclusion and the alleged man is not the biologic father.
C. There is a second-order exclusion and the alleged man is not the biologic father.
D. Insufficient information is given.

320. In the case below, which alleged father is being falsely accused of paternity :

Phenotype

Mother	A19, x; B13, B21
Child	A9, A19; B14, B21
Alleged father 1	A1, A10, B5, B35
Alleged father 2	A9, A28, B18, B14

A. Alleged father 1
B. Alleged father 2
C. Both are being falsely accused based on the results
D. Neither of the above

Ans. **318. A** **319. B** **320. B**

MCQ's ASKED IN VARIOUS ENTRANCE EXAMINATIONS

MCQ's ASKED IN VARIOUS ENTRANCE EXAMS

1. In von Willebrands disease, which is true : **PGI 1986, 91**

A. Normal prothrombin time
B. Decreased platelets
C. Normal partial thromboplastin time
D. All of the above

2. Mode of action of heparin include following, except :
Delhi 1988, 93, 98

A. ↑ Factor-X
B. ↑ Factor-XIII
C. Inhibits thrombin formation
D. Inhibits fibrin formation

3. Following mismatched blood, transfusion all are true, except :
AI 1993, 95, 96

A. Severe reaction possible every after few seconds
B. Pain in back + itching usually feeling
C. ↓ Fibrinolytic activity
D. May present as bleeding

4. In thalassemia not seen is : **Delhi 1988, 95, 97**

A. ↑ Foetal hemoglobin
B. Reduced iron levels
C. Target cells
D. Hb A2 normal or raised

5. Massive blood transfusion causes : **Delhi 1986, 95, 97**

A. Disseminated intravascular coagulation
B. Citrate intoxication
C. Thrombocytopenia
D. Platelet adhesion

6. Serious bleeding occurs if platelet count is below :
Kerala 1994

A. 1,00,000
B. 10,000
C. 60,000
D. 40,000

Ans. 1. A 2. A 3. C 4. B 5. C 6. D

7. **Quick prothrombin time is prolonged in following, except :** **AMU 1988, 92**

A. Factor-V deficiency B. Factor-VII deficiency
C. Vit K deficiency D. AHG deficiency

8. **Helmet cells and other schistocytes are suggestive of :** **AIIMS 1982, 86, 95**

A. Megaloblastic anaemia
B. Iron deficiency anaemia
C. Thalassemia
D. Microangiopathic haemolytic anaemia

9. **In sickle cell anaemia, the pathology may be represented as :** **PGI 1985; Kerala 1987, 95**

A. HbS B Glu-Val B. HbS A 6 Glu-Val
C. HbS B Glu-Val D. Hbs 8 Glu-Val

10. **The osmotic lysis of normal red blood cells begins at a saline concentration of :** **UPSC 1994, 97**

A. 0.6% B. 0.48%
C. 0.36% D. 0.24%

11. **Normal red cell survival time is about :** **UPSC 1985; Delhi 1992,97**

A. 10 days B. 40 days
C. 60 days D. 120 days

12. **HbA_{ic} is :** **AI 1995**

A. A mutant of hemoglobin
B. Absent in 10% normal people
C. Is a result of enzymatic degradation of glucose
D. Indicates levels of glucose in blood

13. **Deficiency of which factor is more likely to be associated with paraproteinemia involving immunoglobulin :** **AIIMS 1984**

A. V B. VII
C. VIII D. XII

14. **Heparin requires for its action :** **PGI 1981**

A. Antithrombin-I B. Antithrombin-III
C. Antithromboplastin D. Antithrombin-VI

15. **Prothrombin time evaluates the activity of following factors except :** **PGI 1982, 88**

A. II B. VII
C. IX D. X

Ans. **7. D** **8. D** **9. A** **10. A** **11. D** **12. D**
13. D **14. B** **15. C**

16. **Following are Vitamin dependent factors, except : PGI 1982, 90**
A. II B. V
C. VII D. IX

17. **The total daily loss of iron amounts to about : PGI 1984, 92**
A. 0.1 mg B. 0.5 mg
C. 1 mg D. 10 mg

18. **First abnormality to appear in iron deficiency anaemia is : AIIMS 1982, 95**
A. Hypochromia B. Microcytosis
C. Elliptocytosis D. Ovalocytosis

19. **Reticulocyte matures into an adult red cells in about : PGI 1980, 86, 94**
A. 2 days B. 3 days
C. 4 days D. 6 days

20. **$\alpha_2\delta_2$ polypeptide chain is present in : AMC 1984, 92**
A. Hemoglobin-A B. Haemoglobin-A_1
C. Haemoglobin-A_2 D. Haemoglobin-S

21. **The minimal amount of methaemoglobin in the blood generally required in order to produce recognisable cyanosis is : PGI 1983, 90**
A. 100 mg B. 250 mg
C. 500 mg D. 1.5 gm

22. **Haemoglobin is characterized by : DNB 1986, 90**
A. Hydrophobic bonding in the reduced state
B. Intracellular crystallization
C. Alpha chain substitution
D. Fast migration at pH 8.6

23. **Normal serum osmolality is : PGI 1988, 96**
A. 250 mosm/kg B. 270 mosm/kg
C. 280 mosm/kg D. 300 mosm/kg
E. 330 mosm/kg

24. **Exchange blood transfusion is indicated in following conditions : Rajasthan 1994, 99**
A. Infants of drug addicts mothers
B. DIC
C. Necrotizing enterocolitis
D. Hereditary fructose intolerance

Ans. **16. B** **17. C** **18. B** **19. A** **20. C** **21. D**
22. B **23. C** **24. A**

25. Packed RBCs are prepared by : **Rajasthan 1996**

A. Filtration B. Centrifugation

C. Distillation D. Electrophoresis

26. Consider the following statements : **CSE 1996, 99**

Disseminated intravascular coagulopathy results in bleeding and is treated by :

1. Replacement of coagulation factors
2. Platelet concentrates
3. Heparin

Of these statements

A. 1, 2 and 3 are correct B. 1 and 2 are correct

C. 1 and 3 are correct D. 2 and 3 are correct

27. Consider the following steps : **UPSC 1997**

1. Whole blood transfusion
2. Granulocyte transfusion
3. Granulocyte monocyte colony stimulating factor
4. Antibiotics

The management of neutropenia (WBC less than 500 cells/microlitre) would include :

A. 1, 2 and 3 B. 2 and 3

C. 2, 3 and 4 D. 1 and 4

28. Hemophilia 'C' is : **PGI 1984**

A. Autosomal dominant B. Autosomal recessive

C. Sex linked recessive D. Sex linked dominant

29. The decrease in hematocrit is vital if it is less than :

AIIMS 1985, 93

A. 40% B. 25%

C. 30% D. 20%

30. Best test for assessing function of platelets is : **AIIMS 1985, 96**

A. Bleeding B. Clotting time

C. Clot retraction time D. Prothrombin time

31. Daily requirement of Vitamin-K in adult is : **PGI 1988, 90**

A. 20-30 microgram

B. 30-50 microgram

C. 70-140 microgram

D. More than 150 microgram

Ans. **25. B** **26. A** **27. C** **28. B** **29. D** **30. C**
31. C

32. **Converging point of both pathways in coagulation is at : PGI 1988, 92**
A. Factor-VIII B. Stuart factor-X
C. Factor-IX D. Factor-VII

33. **Which of the following is not a good screening test for haemorrhagic disease : Kerala 1999**
A. Bleeding time B. Clotting time
C. Prothrombin time D. aPTT

34. **Efficacy of anticoagulant heparin is best monitored by : Kerala 1999**
A. PT B. aPTT
C. FDP level D. Clotting time

35. **True about anemia of chronic disease is : PGI 1999, 2001**
A. ↓ Serum iron, ↑ serum ferritin, ↓ transferrin
B. ↑ Serum iron, ↑ serum ferritin, ↑ transferrin
C. N serum iron, N serum ferritin, N transferrin
D. ↑ Serum iron, ↓ serum ferritin, ↓ transferrin

36. **Plasmapheresis is indicated for which of the following : AIIMS 2001**
A. Wegener's granulomatosis
B. Henoch-Schonlein purpura
C. Goodpasture's syndrome
D. Acute transplant rejection

37. **Drug useful in mild hemophilia is : Delhi 2002**
A. Corticosteroids B. DDAVP
C. Vitamin-K D. Tranexamic acid

38. **One unit of fresh blood raises the Hb% concentration by : AI 2003**
A. 0.1 gm% B. 1 gm%
C. 2 gm% D. 2.2 gm%

39. **Memory T-cells can be identified by using the following marker : AI 2003**
A. CD45RA B. CD45 RB
C. CD45RC D. CD45 RO

40. **Which of the following is a pan-T lymphocytes marker : AI 2003**
A. CD2 B. CD3
C. CD19 D. CD25

Ans. **32. B** **33. B** **34. B** **35. A** **36. A** **37. B**
38. B **39. D** **40. A**

41. Most sensitive and specific test for diagnosis of iron deficiency is : **AI 2003**

A. Serum iron levels
B. Serum ferritin levels
C. Serum transferrin receptor population
D. Transferrin saturation

42. Which of the following marker in the blood is the most reliable indicator of recent hepatitis-B infection : **AIIMS 2003, 2006**

A. HBsAg B. IgG anti - HBs
C. IgM anti - HBc D. IgM anti - HBe

43. Which one of the following platelet counts is usually associated with increased incidence of spontaneous bleeding : **UPSC 2004**

A. Greater than 80,000/mm^3 B. 40,000/mm^3-50,000/mm^3
C. 20,000/mm^3-40,000/mm^3 D. Less than 20,000/mm^3

44. Which of the following is better indicator of need for transfusion : **AIIMS 1985**

A. Urine output B. Haematocrit
C. Colour of skin D. Clinical examination

45. Which of the following cations or anions are significantly bound to proteins: **AIIMS 1986**

A. Magnesium B. Calcium
C. Sodium D. Potassium

46. The most common cause of defective haemostasis is : **Rohtak 1986, 98**

A. Increased fibrinogen B. Anticoagulants
C. Factor-VIII deficiency D. Factor-II deficiency
E. Thrombocytopenia

47. Fresh frozen plasma may be utilized in which of the following deficiencies : **Rohtak 1995**

A. Classical heamophilia B. von Willebrand's disease
C. Factor-V deficiency D. All of the above
E. None of the above

48. The weight of the patient subsisting entirely on parenteral fluids should: **AIIMS 1986, 92**

A. Gain 100 - 200 gm per day.
B. Keep weight steady
C. Loose 100 -200 gm per day
D. Loose 300 - 500 gm per day

Ans. **41.B** **42. C** **43. D** **44. A** **45. B** **46. E**
47. A **48. C**

49. **Following blood which is ready for transfusion is to remain for four hours in a warm environment because it :** **UPSC 1986**

A. Reduces shock

B. Increases shock

C. Favours subsequent hepatitis

D. Encourages bacterial proliferation and septicemia

50. **In an adult, full term infant and preterm baby, blood volumes are ———ml\kg of body weight respecti-vely.** **AIIMS 1984, 90**

A. 70, 80, 90 B. 90, 80, 70

C. 80, 90, 70 D. 90, 70, 90

51. **Signs of hypocalcemia starts appearing when serum levels of ionized calcium falls below:** **Rohtak 1985**

A. 8 B. 7

C. 6 D. 4

52. **Hypoglycemia in full term and preterm babies is defined as blood glucose levels below ———mg/dl respectively.** **AIIMS 1986**

A. 40, 20 B. 20, 40

C. 20, 10 D. 30, 50

53. **Fluid therapy in a patient of shock should begin with :** **UP 1996**

A. Blood transfusion B. Crystalloid infusion

C. Plasma transfusion D. Lomodex infusion

54. **An intravenous infusion for a patient following gastrectomy should include the following anion :** **UP 1996, 2001**

A. Bicarbonate B. Lactate

C. Phosphate D. Chloride

55. **Stored plasma is deficient in :** **DNB 1990**

A. Factors 7 and 8 B. Factors 8 and 9

C. Factors 5 and 8 D. Factors 7 and 9

E. None of the above

56. **Hypokalemia is frequently responsible for which of the following :** **Rohtak 1986**

A. Shortened P-R interval, decrease in P-wave altitude

B. Alkaline urine

C. Paralytic ileus

D. Hyperreflexia

E. Oliguria

Ans. **49. D** **50. A** **51. D** **52. A** **53. B** **54. D**
55. C **56. C**

57. Hypocalcemia is frequently found in which of the following states : Rohtak 1986

A. Hypoproteinaemia
B. Hypoxic acidosis
C. Acute pancreatitis
D. Magnesium depletion
E. All of the above

58. The most effective simple screening test for 'bleeders' is : AMU 1987, 91, 97

A. Peripheral blood smear
B. Whole blood clotting time
C. P.T.T. plus quick test
D. Clot retraction
E. Only A and C

59. Coumarin reversal can best be performed with: Rohtak 1986, 99

A. Blood transfusion
B. Vitamin K_1
C. Vitamin K_2
D. Protamine sulphate
E. Fibrinogen infusion

60. Which of the following routes of cortisol acetate , replacement is least effective : PGI 1984

A. Intramuscular
B. Intravenous
C. Oral
D. Rectal suppository

61. Protein loss after severe trauma occurs because of all of the following, except : AIIMS 1984

A. Starvation
B. Increased catabolism
C. Bed rest
D. Fever
E. None of the above

62. Complications of total intravenous nutrition include which of the following : AIIMS 1985, 88, 96

A. Sepsis
B. Pulmonary embolus
C. Hyperosmolar coma
D. Aortic valve endocarditis
E. All of the above

63. In an acute situation where bleeding is massive and there is no time to type and cross match blood, which of the following should be utilised : PGI 1986, 90

A. Type AB Rh positive blood
B. O Rh positive
C. O Rh negative
D. A Rh negative
E. Ringer's lactate

Ans. 57. E 58. E 59. B 60. A 61. E 62. E 63. C

64. **Which of the following vitamins appear to be essential in postoperative parenteral therapy : PGI 1986**
A. Vitamin-C
B. Vitamin-B
C. Vitamin-D and A
D. Vitamin-D
E. Thiamine

65. **Sudden hypovolemia due to haemorrhage is responsible for release of : PGI 1984, 99**
A. Aldosterone
B. Tryptophan
C. Testosterone
D. Serotonin
E. Thyroxine

66. **Which does not occur in the first week of IV hyperalimentation: PGI 1988; AI 1989, 95**
A. Weight gain
B. Uremia
C. Jaundice
D. Ketosis

67. **Hypovolemic shock manifest when the percentage of blood loss exceeds : AIIMS 1986; AI 1989, 95, 98**
A. 10%
B. 15%
C. 25%
D. 30%
E. 40%

68. **Blood clot of the size of clenched fist is roughly equal to : Delhi 1983**
A. 250 ml
B. 350 ml
C. 500 ml
D. 600 ml

69. **Blood platelets in stored blood do not remain functional after —— hrs. AIIMS 1986**
A. 24
B. 48
C. 72
D. 96

70. **Half life of factor VIII is : AIIMS 1982, 84, 90, 92**
A. 7 hours
B. 18 hours
C. 34 hours
D. 48 hours

71. **In patients subsisting entirely on parenteral fluids, there is daily weight loss of ——. PGI 1981, 88, 97**
A. 50 gm
B. 150 gm
C. 200 gm
D. 250 gm

72. **Following are used in embolism, except : JIPMER 1992, 98**
A. L.V. Heparin
B. Corticosteroids
C. Hyperbaric oxygen
D. Streptokinase

Ans. 64. E 65. A 66. A 67. B 68. C 69. A 70. A 71. B 72. D

73. Reactionary haemorrhage is seen : DNB 1987, 92, 97

A. At the time of operation B. Within 12 hours of operation

C. After more than 10 days D. After more than one month

74. Secondary haemorrhage occurs : AMU 1987, 99

A. Immediately after operation

B. Within one day of operation

C. Within one-to-two weeks of operation

D. Within six months of operation

75. Haematochezia means passage of ———. TN 1996

A. Bloody stools B. Tarry stools

C. Bloody urine D. Bloody bile

76. All of the following are surgical indications of whole blood transfusion, except : PGI 1982, 90

A. During major operative procedure

B. Preoperatively in cases of severe chronic anemia

C. In haemophilic patients before surgery

D. Following severe burns

77. Darrow's solution does not contain : AP 1989, 91

A. Sodium chloride B. Potassium chloride

C. Sodium bicarbonate D. Molar sodium lactate

78. In the immediate post-operative period, body potassium is : AMU 1986, 96

A. Exchanged with calcium

B. Exchanged with magnesium

C. Retained in body

D. Excreted excessively.

79. In the acutely shocked patient, attainment of which of the following is most likely to show adequacy of perfusion of vital organs: AIIMS 1983, 85, 86, 92

A. Normal urine output

B. Normal arterial oxygen tension

C. Normal bicarbonate levels in the blood

D. Normal arterial blood pressure

80. Cryoprecipitate is a rich source of : AIIMS 1985, 92, 99

A. Thromboplastin B. Factor-VIII

C. Factor-X D. Factor-VII

Ans. 73. B 74. C 75. A 76. B 77. C 78. D 79. A 80. B

81. 20 mEq (mmol) of potassium chloride in 500 ml of 5% dextrose solution is given intravenously to treat : **AIIMS 1984, 86**

A. Metabolic alkalosis B. Respiratory alkalosis
C. Metabolic acidosis D. Respiratory acidosis

82. A 45-kg patient presents with BP-70/50 mmHg, Na+ = 115 meq/1. Na+ deficit is to be corrected to 135 meq/L. How many litres of isotonic saline is needed for the patient : **CMC 1998, 91**

A. 13 L B. 18 L
C. 23 L D. 27 L

83. A useful; though temporary improvement in a patient's ischaemic foot can be attained by giving intravenously : **Delhi 1984, 87**

A. 10% Mannitol B. 10% Dextrose
C. Dextran 40 D. Dextran 100

84. Total amounts of fluids to be given within first 24 hours in a patient of 70 kg weight and 40% burns according to Parkland's formula is : **PGI 1986, 88**

A. 11,200 cc B. 7,600 cc
C. 7,000 cc D. 5,500 cc

85. In compatible blood transfusion, all are seen, except : **AIIMS 1986, 93**

A. Bleeding from the wound
B. Thrombophlebitis at the injection site
C. Renal failure
D. Pyrexial reaction

86. In operation theatre tourniquets are used for all of the following conditions, except : **PGI 1982, 85**

A. To control haemorrhage temporarily while exploration and repair has been done.
B. For some amputations.
C. For amputation in arterio sclerotic gangrene.
D. In order to obtain a bloodless field.

87. An overdose of Heparin is treated by : **DNB 1989**

A. Prostaglandins B. Phenindione
C. Protamine sulphate D. Prostigmine

88. Maximum tourniquet time for the upper limb is : **Delhi 1986, 89, 96**

A. 1/2 hour B. 1 hour
C. 1.5 hours D. 2 hours
E. 2.5 hours

Ans. 81. A 82. C 83. C 84. A 85. B 86. C
87. C 88. C

89. While suspecting a blood transfusion reaction, one should :

AMU 1988, 92

A. Continue transfusion of blood and reassess the patient when whole unit of blood has been transfused.

B. Continue transfusion of blood and inject anti-histaminics and steroids.

C. Withdraw the blood transfusion immediately and give injectable antihistaminics and steroids.

D. Inject calcium gluconate immediately.

90. Extracellular fluids losses are often extensive in all, except :

UPSC 1986, 90

A. Hepatic coma B. Peritonitis

C. Intestinal obstruction D. Pancreatitis

91. Of the following which is not the sign of increasing blood loss :

AIIMS 1984, 91

A. Shallow slow breathing

B. Increase pulse rate

C. Increased pallor

D. Restlessness

92. Which of the following would least likely to occur as an untowards reaction to heparin : AIIMS 1985, 93

A. Osteoporosis B. Haemorrhage

C. Hypernatremia D. Respiratory distress

93. The fully developed picture of hypovolemic shock is characterized by the following, except : AIIMS 1985

A. Bradycardia

B. Oliguria

C. Mental dullness

D. Peripheral vasoconstriction

94. The maximum life of a transfused R.B.C. is :

DNB 1989, 92, 95, 99, 2002

A. One hour B. One day

C. 15 days D. 50 days

E. 100 days

95. Haemorrhage is usually well tolerated in a healthy adult upto a maximum of : CSE 1996, 99

A. 500 ml B. 750 ml

C. 5% of blood volume D. 10% of blood volume

Ans. 89. C 90. A 91. A 92. C 93. A 94. E 95. B

96. **Consider the following statements regarding haemorrhagic shock :** **CSE 1997**

1. Normal haematocrit suggests minor bleeding
2. Peripheral vasoconstriction is characteristic
3. Anxiety and sweating are often presents

Of these statements :

A. 1 and 2 are correct B. 1 and 3 are correct
C. 2 and 3 are correct D. 1, 2 and 3 are correct

97. **In a patient on anticoagulant therapy, the INR is maintained at :** **UPSC 2001, 03**

A. 1.5 to 2.5 times of the normal
B. 2.5 to 3.5 times of the normal
C. 3.5 to 4.5 times of the normal
D. 4.5 to 5.5 times of the normal

98. **The percentage of the circulating blood volume in the venous system and splanchnic vessels is normally between :** **AMU 1988**

A. 20-30% B. 40-45%
C. 60-70% D. None of the above

99. **After haemorrhage, lost plasma proteins are replaced by :** **DNB 1989, 93**

A. The small intestine B. The liver
C. The spleen D. The muscles

100. **Ringer lactate contains :** **AIIMS 1985, 86**

A. Na^+, K^+ B. Na^+, K^+, Cl^-
C. Na^+, only D. Na^+, K^+, Cl^-, Ca^+

101. **The anti-coagulant solution commonly used to store blood is :** **AIIMS 1986, 87, 93**

A. Heparin B. EDTA
C. Na-citrate D. Acid citrate dextrose

102. **Blood transfusion reaction during surgery is mediated by :** **JIPMER 1997, 99**

A. Pyrexia
B. Hemetemesis
C. Excessive haemorrhage from the wound site
D. Hypertension

103. **All are complications of IV lipid infusion, except :** **AIIMS 1987, 95**

A. Lactic acidosis B. Ketosis
C. Deterioration of LFT D. Thrombocytopenia

Ans. **96. C** **97. B** **98. C** **99. B** **100. D** **101. D**
102. C **103. D**

104. In a acute trauma, adequate urine output is : **AMC 1985; PGI 1989, 96**

A. 10-15 cc/hour B. 20-30 cc/hour
C. 30-45 cc/hour D. 20-25 cc/hour

105. The decreased in hematocrit is vital if it is less than : AIIMS 1986, 90

A. 40% B. 25%
C. 30% D. 20%

106. The best method to control severe external haemorrhage is : **AIIMS 1983; AMC 1987, 92**

A. Pressure by finger B. Haemostasis
C. Tourniquet to artery D. Tourniquet to vein

107. Fluid replacement is indicated in following types of shoc, except : **NIMHANS 1997, 99**

A. Hypovolemic shock B. Anaphylactic shock
C. Haemorrhagic shock D. Cardiogenic shock

108. The most common hemostatic defect encountered in surgery is : **Karnataka 1993, 98**

A. Christmas disease B. Hemophilia
C. Fibrinolysis D. Thrombocytopenia

109. The volume of the various fluid compartments of the body depends on : **Karnataka 1993, 97**

A. Body size B. Weight
C. Sex D. All of the above

110. The principal buffers of the extracellular fluid space are : **Karnataka 1993, 96**

A. Proteins
B. Phosphates
C. Bicarbonate carbonic acid
D. All of the above

111. Spontaneous bleeding usually occurs with a platelet count of : **Karnataka 1993, 97**

A. Less than 50,000 mm^3 B. 50,000—75,000/mm^3
C. 75,000—1,00,000/mm^3 D. 1,00,000—1,50,000/mm^3

112. Which one of the following factors does not play a role in fluid retention after injury : **UPSC 1994, 96**

A. Antidiuretic hormone B. Capillary permeability
C. Renin D. Hyperglycemia

Ans. **104. C** **105. D** **106. A** **107. D** **108. D** **109. D**
110. D **111. A** **112. A**

113. How long (hours) must a vessel, 1-3.5 mm in diameter, be ligated to produce haemostasis : **DNB 1989, 93**

A. 12 B. 24
C. 48 D. 96

114. Commonest artery for cannulation is : **PGI 1997, 2000**

A. Radial B. Ulnar
C. Brachial D. Femoral

115. The number of calories provided by 3 litres of 5% dextrose solution are : **Delhi 1992, 95**

A. 600 calories B. 1000 calories
C. 1600 calories D. 2000 calories

116. All of the following are causes of increased coagulability of blood except : **PGI 1988**

A. Infections B. After burns
C. Visceral carcinoma D. After haemorrhage

117. Most excessive bleeding occurs when an artery is : **PGI 1995, 97**

A. Completely severed
B. Partially severed
C. Ends are trapped within fracture bone ends
D. Thrombosed

118. Central venous pressure monitoring is helpful in : **UPSC 1997**

A. Regulating the speed and amount of fluid infusion.
B. Regulating the dose of noradrenaline.
C. Deciding the need for plasma infusion.
D. Deciding the requirement for blood transfusion.

119. By which route is the administration of replacement fluid is preferred : **Orissa 1999, 2001**

A. Oral B. Intravenous
C. Intramuscular D. Subcutaneous

120. Consider the following sign(s) : **CSE 1999, 2001**

1. Increasing pallor
2. Restlessness
3. Air hunger
4. Water-hammer pulse

Haemorrhagic shock due to acute blood loss includes :

A. 1 and 4 B. 1 and 2
C. 1, 2 and 3 D. 2, 3 and 4

Ans. 113. D 114. A 115. A 116. B 117. C 118. A 119. C 120. C

121. The best treatment for a patient with dehydration repeated vomiting and having metabolic alkalosis is : AIIMS 1999, 2003

A. NH_4Cl B. I.V. saline
C. I.V. potassium D. I.V. saline + potassium

122. 0.5 Lt. blood loss in 30 min. in normal healthy man produces : AIIMS 1999

A. Increased H.R. with low B.P.
B. Prominently increased H.R.
C. Low B.P., low H.R.
D. Normal B.P. with slightly raised H.R.

123. Ankle brachial pressure index > 1 is seen in : Kerala 1999, 2000

A. Partial obstruction
B. Impending gangrene
C. Normal lower limb vessels
D. Complete obstruction

124. External haemorrhage is initially best controlled by: JIPMER 2000

A. Tourniquet B. Elevation of limb
C. Pressure at the site D. Operative treatment

125. By definition, what percentage loss of blood is termed as severe haemorrhagic shock : DNB 2001

A. Below 20 B. Below 20-40
C. Above 40 D. More than 60

126. Most common haematological abnormality seen in massive blood transfusion is : Kerala 2001

A. Dilutional thrombocytopenia
B. Depletion of factor 5
C. Depletion of factor 8
D. All of the above

127. A person brought to ER with h/o accident 36 hrs back in shock, which is the best method for fluid replacement in this case : Kerala 2001

A. PCV & ESR B. CVP
C. Pulse & BP D. Clinical assessment

128. The most commonly used formula for fluid replacement in the first 24 hours in burns is : Karnataka 1998

A. 2-4 cc/kg. body weight/percentage of burns.
B. 6 cc/kg. body weight/percentage of burns.
C. 8 cc/kg. body weight/percentage of burns.
D. 10 cc/kg. body weight/percentage of burns.

Ans. **121. A** **122. A** **123. C** **124. C** **125. C** **126. A**
127. B **128. A**

129. Wallace's formula of nine for burn is not applicable to the following, except : DNB 1990, 94

A. Children B. Elderly
C. Pregnant females D. Electrical burns

130. The ideal indicator of sufficient fluid replacement in burns is : AIIMS 1983, 85, 88, 89, 93, 99

A. CVP B. Urine output
C. BP D. Arterial wedge pressure

131. Maximum fluid requirement per body area is in: Delhi 1988, 92

A. First week B. 1-4 weeks
C. 4-12 weeks D. 24 weeks

132. In a patient with burns between 25-50% the number of rations to be given in the form of blood is: DNB 1991

A. 4 B. 3
C. 2 D. 1

133. Vasoconstriction in a burns patient fails to maintain the blood pressure when blood loss increases beyond: AIIMS 1982, 86, 90

A. 5-10% B. 10-20%
C. 20-30% D. 50%

134. The best guide to adequate tissue perfusion in the fluid management of a patient with burns, is to ensure a minimum hourly urine output of : Karnataka 2004

A. 10-30 ml. B. 30-50 ml.
B. 50-70 ml. D. 70-100 ml.

135. Acid phosphatase is specific for : AIIMS 2006, 07

A. Monocytes B. Myelocytes
C. B-cells D. T-cells

136. The blood in the vessels normally does not clot because : AI 2004

A. Vitamin-K antagonists are present in plasma.
B. Thrombin has a positive feedback on plasminogen.
C. Sodium citrate in plasma chelates calcium ions.
D. Vascular endothelium is smooth and coated with glycocalyx

137. All the statements about lactoferrin are true, except : AI 2003

A. It is present in secondary granules of neutrophil.
B. It is present in exocrine secretions of body.
C. It has great affinity for iron.
D. It transports iron for erythropoiesis.

Ans. **129. C** **130. B** **131. B** **132. C** **133. C** **134. B**
135. D **136. D** **137. D**

138. A 40 years old male had undergone splenectomy 20 years ago. Peripheral blood smear examination would show the presence of : AIIMS 2003

A. Dohle bodies
B. Hypersegmented neutrophils
C. Spherocytes
D. Howell-Jolly bodies

139. Prothrombin time is a function of all of the following, except : TNPSC 1997

A. Factor-II
B. Factor-V
C. Factor-VII
D. Factor-IX

140. The sequential activation of clotting factors in Phase- I of coagulation is as follows : TNPSC 1997, 2002

A. Factor-XII, Factor-VIII, Factor-XI, Factor-IX
B. Factor-XII, Factor-XI, Factor-IX, Factor-VIII
C. Factor-VIII, Factor-XII, Factor-IX, Factor-XI
D. Factor-IX, Factor-VIII, Factor-XI, Factor-XII

141. Following are the complications of blood transfusion, except : NIMHANS 1997

A. DIC
B. Infections
C. Pyrexia & rigors
D. Hepatitis-A

142. Characteristic features of the anaemia of chronic disorders include, except : TN 1992

A. Normocytic red cells
B. Low plasma iron
C. High TIBC
D. Increased iron in reticulo-endothelial cells
E. Increased plasma copper

143. The macrophages originate from : Bihar 1991

A. Monocytes
B. Tissue cells
C. Giant cells
D. Lymphocytes
E. Foreign body

144. Spherocytes are seen in peripheral smear in all, except: Kerala 1997, 2001

A. Hereditary spherocytosis
B. Hereditary ellipcytosis
C. Hemolytic anaemia
D. Sickle cell anaemia

Ans. **138. D** **139. D** **140. B** **141. D** **142. C** **143. A** **144. D**

145. First Hb to appear in foetal life : **MP 1998, 2002**

A. HbA2 B. HbF
C. HbA D. Gower Hb

146. The activated partial thromboplastin time test is useful for the detection of deficiency of following, except : **DNB 1990**

A. Factor-XI
B. Pre-kallikrein
C. High molecular weight kininogen
D. Factor-VII
E. Factor-XII

147. Hypersegmented polymorph is characteristically seen in : **Rohtak 1987, 96**

A. Infections B. Iron deficiency
C. Folic acid deficiency D. Malignancy

148. Approximately what percentage of transferrin is saturated with iron in the serum of a normal individual : **DNB 1989, 95**

A. 10% B. 33%
C. 50% D. 66%

149. The colour of hemosiderin is : **AP 1991**

A. Black B. Golden yellow
C. Greenish D. Red

150. Coomb's positive hemolysis is seen in : **PGI 1997, 2003**

A. ITP B. SLE
C. TTP D. Dapsone

151. Life span of neutrophil is : **PGI 1977, 80, 86**

A. 6 hours B. 6 days
C. 10 days D. 15 days

152. The best suited anticoagulant for osmotic fragility test is : **AIIMS 1986, 91, 93, 95, 99**

A. Heparin B. EDTA
C. Trisodium citrate D. Potassium oxalate

153. The normal total iron binding capacity is : **UPSC 1988, 93, 97**

A. 0.5-1.0 mg/litre B. 1.5-2.5 mg/litre
C. 1.0-1.5 mg/litre D. 2.5-4 mg/litre

154. Which is not true of Platelet transfusions : **JIPMER 1990, 92**

A. Platelets are effective for 9-10 days
B. Is effective in ITP
C. Effect decreases with repeated usage
D. Are used in DIC

Ans.	**145. B**	**146. D**	**147. C**	**148. B**	**149. B**	**150. B**
	151. C	**152. D**	**153. D**	**154. A**		

155. Following, are features of Thrombus, except : JIPMER 1992

A. Friable B. Easily detached
C. Dry D. Mottled

156. Dithionite test is done for assessing : AMU 1984, 90

A. HbF B. HbE
C. HbA D. HbC
E. HbS

157. All of the following statements about neutrophil granulocytes are true, except : MAHE 1994

A. They are motile.
B. They cannot leave the circulation.
C. They contain lysosomes.
D. They are attracted chemically to sites of inflammation.

158. The average specific gravity of whole blood is : PGI 1980, 85, 93

A. 1.010 B. 1.035
C. 1.055 D. 1.090

159. For whole blood transfusion which of the following is the indication : PGI 1982, 94

A. Acute blood loss
B. Anemia
C. Chronic granulocytic leukaemia
D. Thrombocytopenic purpura

160. For exchange transfusion in haemolytic disease of the new born : AIIMS 1982, 93, 98

A. Fresh blood should be used
B. Only plasma should be used
C. Old blood of 7 days duration can be used
D. All of the above can be used

161. Granules of eosinophils contain all of the following, except : PGI 1982, 94, 95

A. Histaminase B. Phospolipase
C. Aryl sulphatase-B D. Trypsin

162. Hageman factor in clotting is : PGI 1986, 93

A. Factor-III B. Factor-VII
C. Factor-XII D. Factor-VIII

163. A false positive sickling test may be found in : AIIMS 1980, 92

A. Recently transfused blood B. Infected blood sample
C. HbC-Harlem D. All of the above

Ans. **155. B** **156. E** **157. B** **158. C** **159. A** **160. A**
161. D **162. C** **163. D**

164. Mild hemolytic anaemia is associated with vitamin——— deficiency. **AIIMS 1983, 98**

A. B_1 B. E
C. A D. C

165. Lines of Zahn occurs in : **AI 1990**

A. Postmortem clot B. Infarct
C. Embolus D. Coralline thrombus

166. The normal adult blood contains : **AIIMS 1986, 92**

A. Only HbA B. HbA + HbA
C. HbA + HbF D. HbA + HbF + HbA2

167. Bleeding diathesis is a common presenting symptom in : **PGI 1982, 90, 93**

A. Acute promyelocytic Leukaemia
B. Chronic myeloid Leukaemia
C. Myelomonocytic Leukaemia
D. Chronic Lymphoid Leukaemia

168. "Kleihauer test" is used to know : **UPSC 1988, 93**

A. Number of foetal cells in maternal circulation.
B. To find out the deficiency of factor VIII.
C. To find out the exact number of platelets.
D. None of the above.

169. Blood when stored at 4°C can be kept for : **AIIMS 1984, 91**

A. 7 days B. 14 days
C. 21 days D. 28 days

170. Spherocytosis in peripheral blood is not found in : **AIIMS 1988, 93**

A. Thalassemia major
B. Hereditary spherocytosis
C. G-6-P-D deficiency
D. Autoimmune hemolytic anaemia

171. Findings of intravascular hemolysis are, except : **PGI 1987, 91**

A. Increased hemoglobulinuria
B. Increased hemosiderinuria
C. Increased haptoglobulins
D. Hemoglobinemia

172. ESR depends on : **PGI 1987, 92**

A. Viscosity B. Fibrinogen
C. Rouleaux formation D. Verticality of tube
E. All of the above

Ans. **164. B** **165. D** **166. D** **167. A** **168. A** **169. C**
170. C **171. C** **172. E**

173. Test of Hess is done to assess : **Delhi 1983, 93, 95, DNB 1990**

A. Bleeding time B. Capillary fragility
C. Clotting time D. Prothrombin time

174. Prothrombin time is increased in : **AIIMS 1988, 96**

A. Willebrand's disease
B. Afibrinogenemia
C. Qualitative defect of platelets
D. Thrombocytopenia

175. The indirect antiglobulin (Coombs') test is used to : **MAHE 1995**

A. Confirm antibacterial antibodies in the serum.
B. Determine delayed hypersensitivity reactions.
C. Detect "incomplete" (7s) antibody in the serum.
D. Detect red blood cells coated by globulin in vivo.

176. In a normal person, which of the following statement is correct regarding distribution of platelets in the body : **PGI 1990**

A. 70% circulating and 30% in splenic pool.
B. 30% circulating and 70% in splenic pool.
C. 50% circulating and 50% in splenic pool.
D. All the platelets circulates in the peripheral blood.

177. All of the following are needed for clotting, except : **AIIMS 1990, 93**

A. Calcium B. Collagen
C. Platelets D. Local stasis

178. Rewarmed blood may be kept prior to use for : **PGI 1989, 95**

A. 3 minutes B. 30 minutes
C. 3 hours D. All are wrong

179. Deficiency of B-lymphocytes is detected by : **Delhi 1986, 97, 98**

A. Patch test
B. Decrease Immunoglobulins
C. Graft rejection
D. Total leucocytic count

180. Philadelphia chromosome is an example of : **CSE 1998**

A. Balanced translocation B. Deletion
C. Non-dysfunction D. Duplication

181. Common site of haemopoiesis in foetus is : **Delhi 1984, 89, 94**

A. Liver B. Spleen
C. Bone marrow D. Gut

Ans. **173. B** **174. A** **175. C** **176. A** **177. D** **178. B**
179. B **180. A** **181. A**

182. Which of the following is the best source of factor VIII : Karnataka 1998, 2000

A. Fresh blood B. Fresh frozen plasma
C. Cryoprecipitate D. Platelet concentrate

183. Modified cutler method is used to measure : DNB 1988, 92

A. BT B. CT
C. PT D.. ESR

184. ESR is low in the following, except : PGI 1985, 97

A. CHF B. Newborn
C. Polycythemia D. Sickle cell disease
E. Menstruation

185. Linzenmeter is used to measure : AIIMS 1985, 91

A. BT B. CT
C. PTT D. CRT
E. ESR

186. Replacement of red marrow by fatty marrow in bony cavities starts at the age of : AIIMS 1982, 90

A. 1-2 years B. 2-3 years
C. 4-5 years D. 6-7 years

187. Auer rods (reddish, abnormal lysosomes) are usually seen in : AIIMS 1984, 97

A. Lymphocytes B. Neutrophils
C. Monocytes D. Basophilis

188. Which type of immunological reactions involve the Rh incompatibility : Bihar 1991

A. Type-I B. Type-II
C. Type-IV D. Type-V
E. Any of the above depending upon severity

189. Coomb's test (direct) is positive in : Bihar 1988, 91

A. Cold agglutinin B. Warm agglutinin
C. IgM D. IgG

190. Hemophilia-A is due to deficiency of factor : AIIMS 1990; Bihar 1991

A. VII B. VIII
C. IX D. XI
E. XII

Ans. **182. C** **183. D** **184. E** **185. E** **186. C** **187. C**
188. B **189. D** **190. B**

191. An increase in bleeding and clotting time is seen in : **AIIMS 1986, 95, 97**

A. Hemophilia
B. Christmas disease
C. von Willebrand's disease
D. Idiopathic thrombocytopenic purpura

192. In iron deficiency anaemia, true is : **UPSC 1984, 86; AIIMS 1985, 94, 96**

	Serum iron	*Iron binding capacity*
A.	Low	Low
B.	High	Low
C.	Low	High
D.	Low	Normal

193. Reticulocytosis is not seen with : **AIIMS 1994**

A. Hereditary spherolytosis
B. Following acute bleeding
C. Paroxysmal nocturnal haemoglobinuria
D. Anaemia of chronic renal failure

194. In sickle cell anaemia, at pH 8.6 how many bands are seen on chromatography : **Delhi 1995, 97**

A. 2 B. 3
C. 4 D. 5

195. Intrinsic factor of Castle deficiency causes : **AI 1995**

A. Megaloblastic anemia B. Cooley's anemia
C. Pernicious anemia D. Aplastic anemia

196. Target cells are most commonly noted in : **Rajasthan 1989, 90**

A. HbAC B. HbSS
C. HbCC D. HbEE

197. On performing paper electrophoresis of pH 8, 9 the fastest moving haemoglobin is : **AIIMS 1984, 96, 97, 99, DNB 1989, 93**

A. HbH B. Hb Bart's
C. HbS D. HbA

198. Serum does not contain : **Karnataka 1998**

A. Prothrombin B. Calcium
C. Factor-VII D. Factor-IX

Ans. 191. C 192. C 193. D 194. A 195. C 196. C 197. A 198. C

199. "Extramedullary haemopoiesis" means : AIIMS 1982, 90

A. Haemopoiesis occur outside the medulla.
B. Spleen and liver resume haemopoiesis.
C. Expansion of haemopoiesis down the long bones.
D. None of the above.

200. Exudation of plasma and Leucocytes in acute inflammation is from the : AIIMS 1985; PGI 1989, 93

A. Venules
B. Capillaries
C. Arterioles
D. Arterioles and capillaries

201. Which Hb has protective effect on sickling : AIIMS 1981, 93

A. C B. F
C. D D. E

202. Direct Coomb's test is positive in hemolytic anaemia due to : AIIMS 1987, 92

A. Paroxysmal cold hemoglobinuria
B. Paroxysmal nocturnal hemoglobinuria
C. Hereditary spherocytosis
D. Idiopathic thrombocytopenic purpura

203. Normal myeloid erythyroid ratio is : AIIMS 1985, 96

A. 2: 1 B. 1 : 1
C. 3 :1 D. 5 : 1
E. 6 : 1

204. False positive direct Coomb's test may occur in : PGI 1986, 92

A. Penicillin therapy B. Cephaloridine therapy
C. Phenacetin therapy D. All of the above

205. The number of haemoglobin molecules per red blood cell are : PGI 1982, 95

A. 2 million B. 40 million
C. 280 million D. 360 million

206. von Willebrand factor is : West Bengal 1994; JIPMER 2002

A. Platelet aggregator
B. Platelet aggregator inhibitor
C. Plasminogen activator
D. None of the above

Ans. **199. B** **200. B** **201. B** **202. D** **203. C** **204. D**
205. C **206. A**

207. The one state prothrombin time is an index of the function of : **Karnataka 1994**

A. Extrinsic pathways of coagulation
B. Intrinsic pathways of coagulation
C. Platelet function
D. Capillary function

208. Philadelphia chromosome (Ph1) is commonly associated with : **AMU 1989, 93**

A. Chronic lymphatic leukemia
B. Leukemoid reaction
C. Acute monocytic leukemia
D. None of the above

209. For determination of ESR by Westergren method, the only anticoagulant used is : **DNB 1991**

A. EDTA B. Double oxalate
C. Trisodium citrate D. Heparin

210. Serum Iron levels are low in which one of the following conditions : **AMC 1985, 96**

A. Thalassaemia major B. Haemochromatosis
C. Iron deficiency anemia D. Hemophilia

211. Glanzmann syndrome is due to : **PGI 1995**

A. RBC fragility disturbance
B. Neutropenia
C. Platelet dysfunction
D. Pancytopenia

212. Koilocytes are derived from : **PGI 1996**

A. Immature monocytes
B. Mature monocytes
C. Mature mesenchymal cells
D. Small lymphocytes

213. Drepanocyte is a synonym of : **AIIMS 1993, 96, 2002**

A. Burr cell B. Target cell
C. Sickle cell D. Stomatocyte

214. Echinocytes are types of : **AIIMS 1996, 97**

A. RBC's B. Lymphocytes
C. Monocytes D. Platelets

Ans. 207. A 208. D 209. C 210. C 211. C 212. B
213. C 214. A

215. A single pronormoblast gives rise to about ——— mature cells. **DNB 1995, 98**

A. 6 B. 12
C. 16 D. 24

216. Defect in hemorrhagic disease of newborn is in : **AIIMS 1997**

A. Platelet B. Fibrinogen
C. PT D. BT

217. A neonate has TLC 15000; DC———— P35 L40 E7 and metamyelocyte 15%. Find the absolute neutrophil count : **AIIMS 1999**

A. 5250 B. 7500
C. 2250 D. 6000

218. Prothrombin time detects factors : **TN 1999**

A. 8, 9, 10 B. 9, 10, 11, 12
C. 1, 2, 5, 7, 10 D. 11, 12

219. Decrease in Osmotic Fragility causes hemolysis in : **TN 1999, 2001**

A. α thalassemia B. β thalassemia
C. Sickle cell anemia D. Meth. Hemoglobinemia

220. Spherocytosis of RBC's is a common feature in : **PGI 1999**

A. G-6-P-D deficiency B. Sickle cell anemia
C. CML D. ALL

221. HbA2 concentration in thalassemia trait is : **PGI 1999**

A. <1 B. 1-2.5
C. 2.5-3.5 D. >3.5

222. Normal platelet count is found in : **UP 2000**

A. Wiskott-Aldrich syndrome
B. H.S. purpura
C. Immune thrombocytopenia
D. All of the above

223. Hereditary spherocytosis is due to ------- deficiency. **PGI 2000**

A. Spectrin B. Invertin
C. Cytokeratin D. All of the above
E. Mayer-Rokitansky-K.H. syndrome

224. Transfusion of one unit of factor-VIII concentrate will raise the level by : **Karnataka 2000**

A. 1% B. 2%
C. 10% D. 25%

Ans. **215. C** **216. C** **217. A** **218. C** **219. B** **220. A**
221. D **222. B** **223. C** **224. B**

225. β macroglobulin is derived from : DNB 2001

A. B-cells B. T-cells

C. Both of the above D. None of the above

226. Tissue thromboplastin activates : DNB 2001

A. Factor-VII B. Factor-IV

C. Factor-VI D. None of the above

227. Bleeding tendency start to occur below platelet count : Rohtak 2001, 2004

A. 20,000 B. 40,000

C. 1 lakh D. 2 lakhs

228. Best stain to demonstrate sideroblasts in bone marrow: JIPMER 2002

A. Pearls stain B. Halls stain

C. Fontanna stain D. Weight stain

229. Deficiency of which of the following factors does not cause an abnormality of the intrinsic pathway : SGPGI 2002

A. Factor-IX B. Factor-VII

C. Factor-XI D. Factor-VIII

230. Levels of Hb required to maintain good body growth and normal activities in beta-thalassemic patient is : Maharashtra 2000

A. 6-8 gm% B. 8-10 gm%

C. 10-12 gm% D. > 12 gm%

231. Rouleaux formation can occur after the infusion of : BHU 2002

A. Dextran 40 B. Dextran 70

C. Gelatin D. Human albumin

232. CD-10 is seen in : BHU 2002

A. ALL B. CLL

C. HCL D. CML

233. A 55-years old male, accident victim in casualty urgently needs blood. The blood bank is unable to determine his ABO group, as his red cell group and plasma group, do not match. Emergency transfusion of patient should be with : AIIMS 2002

A. RBC corresponding to his red cell group and colloids/crystalloid.

B. Whole blood corresponding to his plasma group.

C. O-positive RBC and colloids/crystalloid.

D. AB negative whole blood.

Ans. **225. A** **226. A** **227. A** **228. A** **229. B** **230. C**
231. B **232. A** **233. B**

234. Although, more than 400 blood groups have been identified, the ABO blood group system remains the most important in clinical medicine because : **AIIMS 2002**

A. It was the first blood group system to be discovered.
B. It has four different blood groups A, B, AB, O (H).
C. ABO (H) antigens are present in most body tissues and fluids.
D. ABO (H) antibodies are invariably present in plasma when persons RBC lacks the corresponding antigen.

235. Consider the following statements :
Factor-VIII (AHF) is involved in coagulation mechanism of haemostasis : **UPSC 2002**

1. Only in extrinsic pathways
2. Only in intrinsic pathways
3. In common pathways

Which of these statements is/are correct :

A. 1 only B. 2 only
C. 1 and 3 D. 2 and 3

236. The preservative used for storing blood for transfusion is : **AIIMS 1992, 95, 97**

A. CPD-A B. Heparin-dextrose
C. Citrate + glucose D. EDTA

237. At what stage of erythropoiesis does hemoglobin appear : **AIIMS 1992, 99**

A. Early normoblast B. Intermediate normoblast
C. Reticulocyte D. Erythroblast

238. How long can blood be stored with CPD-A : **JIPMER 1993**

A. 21 days B. 28 days
C. 35 days D. 42 days

239. Nonspecific esterase is present in : **PGI 1997**

A. Monocytic leukemia B. Lymphocytic leukemia
C. Erythroleukemia D. All of the above

240. Blood group antigen : **Punjab 1997**

A. Found attached to Hb molecule
B. Found in plasma proteins
C. Sometimes found in saliva
D. Found in bone marrow

Ans. 234. D 235. B 236. A 237. B 238. C 239. A
240. C

241. Left shifting of neutrophils is seen in : **WB 2007**

A. Adenocarcinoma small intestine
B. Liver disease
C. Pheochromocytoma
D. Insulinoma

242. All of the following are antigen presenting cells, except : **AI 2008**

A. Langerhans cells
B. Dendritic cells
C. T-cells
D. Activated B-cells

243. Function of CD4 is all except : **AI 2009**

A. Memory
B. Immunoglobin production
C. Activation of macrophages
D. Cytotoxicity

244. Which of the following drugs will prevent platelet aggregation : **AMC 1999**

A. Paracetamol
B. Sulfonamides
C. I.N.H.
D. Aspirin

245. A positive coomb's test in absence of haemolysis, may be seen with administration of : **UPSC 1995**

A. Cephalothin
B. Ampicillin
C. Nalidixic acid
D. Carbenicillin

246. Major indication for intrauterine transfusion of foetus is : **AIIMS 1982, 92**

A. Bradycardia and foetal distress
B. Sickle cell anaemia
C. Erythroblastosis foetalis
D. None of the above

247. Most common complication of intrauterine transfusion is : **PGI 1983, 99**

A. Graft versus host reaction
B. Premature onset of labour
C. Transfusion reaction
D. None of the above

248. Breakdown of 1 gm of haemoglobin yields about : **AIIMS 1986, 90**

A. 20 mg bilirubin
B. 35 mg bilirubin
C. 5 mg bilirubin
D. 1 mg bilirubin

Ans. **241. B** **242. D** **243. B** **244. D** **245. A** **246. C** **247. C** **248. B**

249. Hazards of exchange transfusion include following, except : **AIIMS 1993, 96**

A. Oligaemic shock B. Citrate tetany
C. Cardiac arrest D. Hypokalaemia

250. Foetal blood in the maternal circulation is detected by : **AIIMS 1982, 88, 90; Delhi 1983; ESI 1994**

A. Hemoglobin estimation B. Optic density
C. Spectrophotometer D. Kleihauer test

251. Hypertransfusion in Thalassemia is given by : **Delhi 1990, 94**

A. 6 gm% B. 8 gm%
C. 10 gm% D. 12 gm%

252. The type of blood to use if time does not permit adequate cross-matching in an emergency is : **AMU 1995, 98**

A. O, Rh negative B. O, Rh positive
C. B, Rh positive D. A, Rh negative

253. Physiologic anemia of newborn is most severe at the age of : **Rohtak 1999, 2002**

A. 4 months B. 2 months
C. 4 weeks D. 2 weeks

254. Haemorrhagic disease of the newborn most commonly appears in : **AP 1999**

A. Haemophilic diseased infants
B. Thrombocytopenic infants
C. Breast-fed infants
D. Early artificial milk-fed infants

255. Serum iron is raised in : **AIIMS 1995**

A. Chronic renal failure B. Thalassemia
C. Iron deficiency anaemia D. Viral hepatitis

256. Haemoglobin- F is : **PGI 1998**

A. a_2b_2 B. a_2g_2
C. a_2d_2 D. a_1b_1

257. 'Warm' type of hermolytic anaemia is caused by all, except : **PGI 1994**

A. Mycoplasma
B. Methyldopa
C. Leukemia (chronic lymphatics)
D. Hodgkin's lymphoma
E. SLE

Ans. **249. D** **250. D** **251. C** **252. A** **253. B** **254. C**
255. B **256. B** **257. A**

258. Foetal acidosis in pH less than : **Rajasthan 1998**

A. 7.0 B. 7.2
C. 7.3 D. 7.4

259. The Hb to appear first in the fetus is : **TN 1993**

A. HbA B. HbA2
C. HbF D. Hb Gower

260. The major site of active haemopoiesis in a foetus of 5 months is : **TN 1993**

A. Spleen B. Liver
C. Lymph nodes D. Bone marrow

261. The percentage of foetal haemoglobin at birth is : **Bihar 1999**

A. 90% B. 20%
C. 70% D. 100%

262. Large doses of Vitamin-K administered to a new-born may result in : **AIIMS 1992**

A. Hypothyroidism B. RBC destruction
C. Bulging of fontanelles D. Prolonged bilirubinemia

263. Philadelphia chromosome is : **AP 1993**

A. t (8; 22) B. t (8; 21)
C. t (15; 17) D. t (8; 14)

264. Sickling of red blood cells occurs in : **PGI 1993**

A. 8% of whites
B. Megaloblastic anemia
C. Only in sickle cell anemia, not sickle cell trait
D. Thalassemia and sickle cell trait occurring together

265. In alpha-thalassemia, HbH is formed by chains of——. **DNB 1990**

A. a_3, b_1 B. a_4
C. a_1, b_3 D. b_4

266. Normal infant has ——— mg of iron at the time of birth: **DNB 1991**

A. 100—200 B. 250—300
C. 500—600 D. 900—1000

267. The following are the correct facts in relation to haemorrhage disease of new born, except : **Karnataka 1999**

A. Self- limited bleeding disorder.
B. Results from deficiency of coagulation factors dependent on Vitamin-K.
C. More common in formula fed infants.
D. In most cases, haemorrhagic manifestations become evident for the 2nd and 3rd day of life.

Ans. **258. B** **259. C** **260. B** **261. C** **262. D** **263. A**
264. D **265. D** **266. B** **267. A**

268. Indication for exchange transfusion at birth is : **Delhi 1995**

A. Cord Hb < 16 gm%

B. Cord bilirubin —3 mg%

C. Cord bilirubin —5 mg%

D. Mother antibody titre > 1 : 64

269. Coomb's positive hemolytic anemia occurs in : **PGI 1999**

A. SLE B. ITP

C. CML D. Rifampicin intake

270. Fetal Hb equals adult Hb at : **TN 1999**

A. Birth B. 2 months

C. 4 months D. 6 months

271. Serum Iron level in child ______ mgm. **TN 1999**

A. 20-50 B. 100-200

C. 50-100 D. 200 - 350

272. In ABO hemolytic disease of the newborn direct Coomb's test is : **UPSC 1984, 87, 92, 95**

A. Usually negative

B. Usually mild positive

C. Usually strongly positive

D. Positive in cases where peripheral smear shows microspherocytosis

273. O +ve mother delivers A -ve baby. Which of the following blood will be ideal if the baby needs exchange blood transfusion : **Rohtak 1984, 97**

A. O -ve

B. A +ve

C. A -ve

D. O -ve cells suspended in AB plasma

274. When does switch over from fetal to adult hemoglobin synthesis begin : **AI 2005**

A. 14 weeks gestation B. 30 weeks gestation

C. 36 weeks gestation D. 7-10 days postnatal

275. Adult hemoglobin at birth is ——— %. **Delhi 2000**

A. 10 B. 20

C. 30 D. 80

Ans. 268. C 269. A 270. B 271. D 272. A 273. D
274. A 275. B

GLOSSARY

GLOSSARY

Abbreviated crossmatch : An immediate-spin saline major crossmatch used to determine ABO compatibility in patients with no demonstrable clinically significant antibodies and a negative history of antibody formation.

Acanthocytosis : Abnormal red cell morphology characterized by cytoplasmic projections resembling thorns.

Acid-citrate-dextrose (ACD) : An anticoagulant/preservative containing citric acid, sodium citrate, and dextrose. ACD whole blood has a shelf life of 21 days. ACD is no longer used for the collection of donor blood because solutions are available that allow for extended shelf life. Owing to the acid pH, 2.3-DPG levels are not well maintained in this solution.

Adaptive Immunity : The ability of the immune system to specifically respond to antigenic challenge, that is, the ability to discriminate between self and non-self. Adaptive immunity can be divided into cellular and humoral immunity.

Adsorption : The attachment of specific antibody to the red cell surface via binding with specific antigen. For example, A cells adsorb anti-A from solution, Adsorption is a blood bank technique in which cells and plasma are mixed, and antibody is adsorbed into the red cell surface.

Affinity : The degree of fit between an antigen and antibody.

Agglutination : The clumping together of antigen bearing cells (such as red blood cells) in the presence of specific antibody.

Albumin : A protein-potentiating agent that enhances the reactions of some clinically significant alloantibodies. Albumin reagents such as 22 per cent, 30 per cent, and polymerized bovine albumin are available commercially.

Alleles : Alternate forms of a gene which can occupy a given chromosomal location (locus). Each individual inherits an allele from the mother and one from the father, making up a homologous pair for each trait.

Allogenic (homologous) transfusion : The transfusion of blood and blood components to individuals other than self (nonautologous).

Allogenic antigens : Antigens that are from the same species but are antigenically distinct. Blood group antibodies can be formed when an individual receives red cells from another individual which carry allogenic antigens. Antibodies made to these alloantigens are known as alloantibodies.

American Association of Blood Banks (AABB) : The professional organization for practitioners in the field of transfusion medicine. The AABB provides standards of excellence for transfusion medicine practice and has a voluntary inspection and accreditation program.

2-aminoethyllsothlouronlum bromide (AET) : A substance capable of inactivating the Kell antigens on the surface of the red cell, rendering the cell Kell null.

Amorph type Rh : A phenotype resulting fromt he inheritance of two r genes.

Anamnestic (secondary) response : The immune response to a second or subsequent exposure to a specific antigen. This response differs in a number of ways from the typical firs : (primary) response.

Anaphylactic reaction : A severe immunologic response to transfusion that is both rapid and life-threatening. Systemic anaphylaxis produces changes in circulation and bronchioles consistent with shock. Anaphylactic reactions cannot be predicted by routine pretransfusion testing.

Anaphylaxis : An allergic reaction to foreign substances associated with fever, redness of the skin, itching, urticaria, dyspnea, chest constriction, cyanosis, irregular pulse, convulsions, hypotension, and death.

Antisocytosis : Abnormal red cells morphology characterized by marked variation in red cell rize.

Antibodies : Immunoglobulin molecles that are produced in response to stimulatin by specific antigen and are capable of combining with the antigen that elicited their production.

anticoagulant/preservative : A solution that is designed to preserve the viability and function of hte collected blood (preservative) and prevent clotting (anticoagulant). Such solutions provide buffering capability and nutrients for cellular metabolism during storage.

Antigen : A substance capable of eliciting an immune response and reacting specifically with the product of that response.

Antigenic determinant/epitope : That portion of the antigen molecule with which antibody can combine.

Antiglobulin phase : The phase of in vitro testing that uses anti-human globulin reagent to detect in vivo or in vitro inding of IgG or complement to red cells.

Antiglobulin technique : The use of anti-human globulin reagents to detect red cell-bound antibodies. This technique is required by the AABB in routine pretransfusion testing. Refer to antiglobulin phase.

Apheresis : The process of removing whole blood from a donor or patient, processing the blood so as to separate selected elements, and returning the unharvested portion to the donor/patient. Apheresis can be cytapheresis, in which cellular components are harvested, or plasmapheresis, in which plasma is harvested.

Arteriovenous fistula : An abnormal direct communication between an artery and a vein.

Autologous : Refers to self components. For example, a transfusion of one's own cells is an autologous transfusion.

Autologous control (autocontrol) : A control with the patient's own serum and cells run in parallel with antibody detection and compatibility testing.

Autosomal inheritance : Inheritance via alleles that are carried on any autosome (except the X or Y sex chromosomes).

Avidity : The strength of the bond between an antigen and its respective antibody.

Azurophillic : The ability to stain with blue analine dyes.

α-2-i fucosyltransferase : the product of the H-gene which transfers fucose to type II chains on the red cells to produce H antigen.

B lymphocytes (B cells) : The precursors of antibody producing plasma cells which are involved primarily in humoral immunity. B-cell maturation takes place predominantly in the bone marrow, and the cells are characterized by the presence of surface immunoglobulin.

Bg antigens : HLA antigens present on red cells which may cause weak and variable reactions with sera containing the corresponding antibody. These antibodies may interfere with the interpretation of pretransfusion antibody detection and identification and may be present as contaminating antibodies in commercial antisera.

Blood center/blood bank : A facility that is generally responsible for all activities that lead to the preparation of suitable blood products for transfusion, including such areas as donor recruitment, phlebotomy, processing, storage, and shipment.

Blood/components request forms : The form issued to initiate the preparation of blood and/or components for a patient. This form must contain the following minimum information: first and last name of the patient and the patient's identification number.

Blood sample label : A label completed and attached in the sample before leaving the patient's bedside. This label must contain the following minimum information; patient's name, patient's identification number, and date of collection. There must also be a mechanism to determine who drew the specimen.

Blood transfusion form : A form completed for each unit of crossmatched blood which contains the following minimum information: patient's name and identification number, ABO and Rh type of the recipient and the donor, donor unit number, pool number (if applicable), interpretation of compatibility testing, and identification of the person performing the tests.

Blood warmers : Devices that warm blood to 37°C inline during infusion.

Bombay phenotype : The rare inheritance of two H genes at the Hh locus and the subsequent lack of the H-antigen. Such individuals are unable to express other ABO antigens.

Bradykinin : A polypeptide substance capable of inducing hypotension, increasing the permeability of capillaries, and eliciting pain.

Cardiopulmonary resuscitation (CPR) : Techniques aimed at the delivery of oxygen to the heart and other vital organs until normal heart and pulmonary function can be restored. All blood center and blood bank personnel should be trained and currently certified to perform CPR.

Catecholamines : the biologically active amines (epinephrine and norepinephrine), which have a marked effect on the cardiovascular system, temperature, and smooth muscle, producing vasoconstriction and smooth muscle relaxation.

Cellular immunity : Immun responses mediated by T-lymphocytes either as a result of direct cytotoxicity or through the liberation of lymphokines.

Chemically modified reagents : Antibodies that have been modified chemically in order to enhance their ability to detect red cell antigens.

Chimera : An individual who has more than one cell population from different sources. In the blood bank, chimerism may result in multiple red cell populations with differing antigens and in discrepant antigen typing results.

Chloroquine diphosphate : A reagent that dissociates IgG from the red cell membrane while maintaining membrane integrity. This technique is useful for removing bound antibody so that cells can be typed for antigens requiring the indirect antiglobulin phase of testing such as Fy.

Chronic granulomatous disease (CGD) : An inherited disorder in which polymorphonuclear leukocytes are able to phagocytize but not to kill certain microorganisms. The disease is characterized by chronic severe bacterial infections.

Circular of Information for the Use of Human Blood and Blood Products : A publication required for all blood and blood products. This pamphlet, which must be available in the transfusion service center, contains information regarding product indications, dosages, side effects, risks, and contraindications.

Citrate-phosphate-dextrose (CPD) : A preservative solution containing citrate, phosphate, and dextrose which, because of its more alkaline pH, more effectively maintains 2,3-DPG levels in stored red cells. CPD red cells can be stored for 21 days. The addition of adenine to CPD (CPDA-1) extends the shelf life of 35 days.

Class-I genes : Alleles at the HLA-A, B, and C loci which are defined (serologically) by complement-dependent cytotoxic reactions using known antisera from immunized humans and monoclonal sources.

Class-II genes : Alleles at the HLA-D locus which are defined by the mixed lymphocyte culture technique.

Class-III genes : Alleles of the major histocompatibility complex which produce a number of functionally diverse molecules.

Clinically significant antibodies : Red cell alloantibodies that react at 37° C and are capable of causing decreased survival or transfused red cells.

CMV-negative : Negative for the antibody to cytomegalovirus (CMV). CMV-negative blood is preferred for immunocomprised recipients to decrease the risk of infection.

Code of Federal Regulations (CFR) : A publication of the Food and Drug Administration which includes regulations pertaining to the manufacture of blood, blood components; and blood products.

Co-dominant traits : Inherited traits that are both expressed whether the allele is present in the homozygous or heterozygous form.

Cold hemagglutinin disease : A condition resulting from the agglutination of red blood cells by a cold-reacting autoantibody. The disease is associated with hemolytic anemia and/or obstruction of the microcirculation.

College of American Pathology (CAP) : A professional organization for clinical pathologists and clinical laboratory scientists. CAP develops standard of practice for clinical laboratories and has a voluntary inspection and accreditation program.

Colloid solutions : A solution with particles too large to pass through animal membranes. Colloids therefore remain in the vasculature and exert an oncotic effect, drawing water into the vascular space. Colloids are indicated for volume expansion.

Compatibility label : a firmly attached unit label that contains the following mainimum information: recipient's name and identification number, donor number, interpretation of compatibility testing, and identification of the person performing the tests.

Compatibility testing : All serologic testing and clerical checks involved in determining compatibility between a potential recipient and donor. Compatibility testing policies are based on prevailing standards of practice and ensure a high probability of a successful transfusion outcome but cannot guarantee safety.

Complement component : An individual element of the complement system, a functionally related group of atleast 20 serum proteins which cause immune cytolysis and other biologic activities.

Complement fixation tests : Laboratory procedures that use complement fixation and resultant cell lysis as an end point.

Component : A product made from the source product whole blood. Components are broken into two general classes: cellular products and plasma products.

Compound antigens : A distinct antigen formed when two additional antigens are produced by the same gene.

Confidential unit exclusion : The opportunity for a blood donor to indicate in confidence that the donated unit should not be used for transfusion. In such cases, all donor testing is completed and the donor is notified of any abnormal results and offered any necessary counselling.

Constant and variable domains or regions : Portions of the immunoglobulin molecule that have constant amino acid sequenced. Those with variable amino acid sequences are known as variable regions. Portions of the variable regions have extreme variability. These hypervariable regions give the antibody molecule its specificity for a particular antigen.

Cooperativity : The condition in which the oxygenation of one heme affects the oxygen affinity of the hemoglobin molecule. This is due to a stearic change in the molecule which occurs when oxygen is gained or lost. Uptake of oxygen increases affinity, whereas release of oxygen decreases affinity.

Cordocentesis : The technique of sampling blood from the fetus in utero.

Critical titer : That titer which at or below no severely affected infants or stillbirths have been reported. Determination of this value is based upon data from the institution. If no data are available, a titer of 32 is often used as a benchmark.

Crossover : The process of placing unused predeposit autologous units into the homologous blood supply.

Cross-reactive groups (CREGS) : Groups of antigens based on their common reactivity with antibodies to public epitopes.

Cross-reactivity : The reactivity of antibodies that have a broad specificty and may react with more than one antigenic determinant or epitope.

Cryoprecipitate/antihemophilic factor (AHF) : The cold-insoluble portion of plasma. The component is rich in Factor VIII-C, von Willebrand factor, Factor XIII, fibrinogen, and fibronectin. This component is indicated for patients with von Willebrand's disease, Factor XIII deficiency obstetrical accidents, and hemophilia A.

Cryoprotective agent : A chemical agent, such as glycerol, capable of protecting cells from freeze injury.

Cryptantigen : An antigen hidden from detection on normal red cells.

Crystalloid solution : A solution that can be diffused through animal membranes. Crystalloids such as normal saline can be used to restore blood volume up to approximately 20 per cent blood loss.

Cyanosis : Bluish discoloration of the skin due to decreased oxygen saturation of the blood.

Cyclosporine : A cyclic polypeptide immunosuppressant agent. Cyclosporine has been shown to inhibit cell-mediated immune reactions, such as allograft rejection, by suppressing the function of T -cells, especially T-helper cells. Cyclosporine is used to prevent graft rejection in kidney, liver, heart, and bone marrow transplant recipients.

Cytoagglomeration : A procedure that causes cells to form reversible masses or clumps.

Cytomegalovirus (CMV) : One of a group of herpesviruses transmitted by the viable leukocytes in blood components which is of special concern when transfusing immunocompromised recipients. Leukodepletion of components and the transfusion of CMV-negative blood are methods of reducing risk.

D-deletion phenotypes : Phenotypes that lack many Rh antigens and may result when some of the Rh genetic material is missing.

α-galactosyltransferase : Transfers the sugar α-galactose to the H antigen, conferring B blood group specificity.

Deglycerolized red blood cells : A component prepared by thawing and washing red cells that have been stored in a cryoprotective agent for extended storage of upto 10 years. This freezing process is especially useful for rare blood storage.

Defense : Immunologically mediated resistance to infection.

Delayed hemolytic transfusion reaction : Accelerated destruction of transfused red cells, usually associated with an anamnestic antibody response to alloantigen(s) on donor red cells. These reactions may not be recognized for days or weeks after transfusion. Anti-2k is frequently associated with delayed hemolytic events. Because delayed reactions are often asymptomatic, many may go unreported.

Density gradient sepatation : A technique used for the separation of particles or cells based on their differential densities. Chemical gradients of known density are used to separate cells into layers during centrifugation.

Desmopressin : An analogue of vasopressin which is used for the management of patients with mild hemophilia A and von Willebrand's disease.

Desquamation : Sloughing of skin.

Diastolic pressure : That period of least pressure in the arterial system which corresponds to the time in the heart cycle when fibers lengthen and the heart dilates and fills (diastole).

Diethylthreltol (DTT) : A thiol reagent that inactivates the Kell antigens (except for K) on the red cell surface. DTT also inactivates CArtwright, LW, and Dombrock system antigens as well most antigens with HTLA characteristics.

Differential centrifugation : The separation of components of differing densities by centrifugation. This technique is used for most blood components preparation.

Dilutional coagulopathy : Dysfunction of hemostasis due to the dilution of coagulation factors and platelets during the massive administration of blood, components, and derivatives.

Dimethyl sulfoxide (DMSO) : A cryoprotective agents used to protect cells from damage during the freezethaw process.

Diploid : The condition of having two sets of chromosomes (maternal and paternal). The somatic cells of higher organisms are diploid.

Direct antiglobulin test (DAT) : A one-step test used to identify red blood cells that have been sensitized with antibody or complement in vivo.

Direct or first order exclusion : Exclusionof paternity because of inheritance by a child of a trait that neither parent possesses.

Directed donation : The process by which donors designate specific recipients for their donated blood and blood components.

Disseminated intravasuclar coagulation (DIC) : A condition associated with the activation of coagulation cascade within the vasculature. DIC causes fibrin deposition in the microcirculation and consumption of platelets and fibrinogen. The major complication of DIC is clinical bleeding.

Dolichos bifloris : A lectin with anti-A, specificity.

Dominance : Inheritance in which a trait is fully expressed when the allele is present in either the homozygous or heterozygous form.

donor screening : The process used to ensure that a potential donation is not harmful in any way to the donor and that the final product(s) provide maximum benefit to the intended recipient. Donor screening involves and inteview and a mini-physical examination.

Dyspnea : Shortness of breath

Edema : A general term for the accumulation of fluid in the tissues.

Electromechanical infusion devices (Infusion pumps) : Devices that control the flow of intravenous fluids.

Elution : The process by which adsorbed antibody (on the red cells surface) is removed and returned to solution. Elutions can be performed by a number of physical and chemical procedures.

Enhancement : Strengthening antibody antigen reactions through a variety of chemical and nonchemical techniques. The most convenient and least expensive of these techniques involve no special reagents or equipments, such as increasing serum-cell ratio.

Enteric, parenteral nutrition, and hyperalimentation : The administration of nourishment through a variety of routes (enteral small intestine; parenteral; sub-cutaneous/intramuscular) or greater than optimal (hyper) amounts.

Enzyme methods : The use of proteolytic enzymes in in vitro tes systems in order to facilitate antibody identification.

Epinephrine : A hormone produced by the adrenal medulla which can be used as a vasoconstrictor and bronchiole dilator.

Equivalence : Optimal antigen-antibody concentrations that facilitate the development of visible agglutination.

Erythema : Redness of the skin caused by capillary dilatation.

Erythroblastosis fetalis : A synonym for hemolytic disease of the newborn. The hemolytic disease is associated with anemia, jaundice, splenomegaly, edema and the presence of immature red cells in the circulation (erythroblasts).

Erythroderma : Widespread erythema.

Erythropoietin : A hormone produced predominantly by the kidneys in response to hypoxia.

Exchange transfusions : The simultaneous withdrawal of blood and infusion of compatible donor blood to infants with hemolytic disease of the newborn. The procedure removes antigen-positive cells, provides cells that are compatible with maternal antibodies, decreases bilirubin levels, and corrects anemia.

Exogenous/endogenous : Exogenous refers to outside and endogenous refers to within. An endogenous disease, for example, arises from circumstances within the organism.

Expiration date : The last date on which stored blood can be used for transfusion. Storage periods are based on in vivo viability standards.

Extended panel : Any panel of antibody identification cells in which the user has selected additional cells for the purpose of clarifying or confirming antibody identification data, such as addition of a A_1, A_2, and cord cells for cold-autoantibody identification.

Extramedullary erythropoiesis : Production of red cells outside of the bone marrow.

Extravascular hemolysis : The premature removal of incompatible transfused red cells from the circulation by the phagocytic cells of the reticuloendothelial system (liver and spleen).

Factor VIII concentrate : A lyophilized commercial product that contains Factor VIII : C and is prepared from the fractionation of plasma. The product is treated of reduce the risk of viral transmission and is indicated for the management of hemophilia A.

Factor IX concentrate : A commercial product similar to Factor-IX complex except that it is more highly purified and the final concentration of Factor-IX is 30 per cent. Both products are indicated for the management of Factor-IX deficiency.

Factor IX complex (prothrombin complex) : A commercial lyophilized product containing Factors II, VII, IX and X . Factor IX makes up about 5 per cent of this product.

Factor XII/Hageman factor : A serine protease (molecular weight 80,000) in the intrinsic coagulation pathway. Factor-XII activation during the process of immune hemolysis contributes to both intravascular coagulation and activation of the kinin system.

Fetal lung maturity : A measure of the ability to inflate alveolar spaces and allow oxygen transport to red blood cells which is related to the production of pulmonary surfactant (lipids). Lung maturity is often monitored using the lecithin/sphingomyelin (L/S) ratio. Others tests for fetal lung maturity include phosphatidylglycerol.

Fetal-maternal hemorrhage : The passage of red cells from the maternal to the fetal circulation due to placental trauma or at delivery.

Fibrin glue : The combination of thrombin and cryoprecipitate used topically to arrest surgical bleeding.

Fisher's exact test : A statistical analysis applied to blood bank antibody identification in order to achieve 95 per cent confidence that the result is valid.

Fresh blood : Whole blood or red cells selected for transfusion early (generally in less than 7 days) within the storage period in order to minimize the infusion of cellula breakdown products and metabolic waste and optimize levels of red cells 2,3-DPG and ATP.

Fresh frozen plasma : Plasma separated from whole blood within 8 hours of donation and frozen at 18°C or below. The process preserves levels of stable and labile coagulation factors for the storage period of 1 year and is indicated in bleeding patients with multiple factor deficiencies.

Frozen red cells : Red cells from whole blood donation separated and frozen within 6 days of donation. Freezing allows for extended storage and is especially valuable for rare blood stockpiling.

Gene : Composed of deoxyribonucleic acid (DNA) genes are the basic unit of inheritance.

Genotype : The genetic make-up of an individual.

Ghost cells : Cells that appear pale and unstained.

Glucose-6-phosphate dehydrogenase deficiency : A deficiency of an enzyme in the pentose pathways associated with hepatomegaly, hypoglycemia, acidosis, decreased serum haptoglobin, and failure to thrive.

Glycophorin A (MN, SGP, PAS-1 PAS-2): A sialoglycoprotein produced by the MNgene.

Glycophorin-B (Ss SGP, PAS-3) A sialoglycoprotein produced by the Ssgene.

Glycosylated : Chemically linked with glycosyl (sugar) groups.

graft-versus-host disease (GVHD): The pathologic reaction resulting from engraftment of donor immuno-component tissue into an immuno compromised host.

Granulocytes : Leukocyte concentrates prepared from a single donor by apheresis techniques. The component contains granulocytes, variable amounts of lymphocytes, platelets, and red cells suspended in approximately 250 ml. of plasma and is indicated for patients with overwhelming sepsis and insufficient numbers of circulating neutrophils.

Granulopoietic factors : Naturally occurring lypoproteins that stimulate the development of granulocytes (granulocytopoiesis).

Group compatible (type compatible) Refers to blood/components in which the product transfused is compatible with (but not identical to) the type of the recipient. If, for example, a unit of red cells is needed for a group-A recipient, group-O cells are suitable because they are compatible with the serum of the recipient.

Group specific (type specific): Refers to blood/components of the identical type as that of the recipient. When transfusing whole blood, type-specific blood must be used.

Haploid : The condition of having one set of chromosomes (maternal or paternal). The sex cells (gametes) of higher organisms are haploid.

Haplotype : A set of alleles from a group of closely linked genes that are inherited together and responsible for the production of a number of blood group antigens. The major antigens of the Kell blood group system, for example, are inherited as haplotypes.

Haptoglobin : A mucoprotein which binds hemoglobin that has been released from lysed red cells. Haptoglobin is decreased in hemolytic disorders.

Hematoma : A mass of blood (usually clotted) which is confined to local region and usually results from the rupture of a blood vessel.

Hemochromatosis : The infiltration of iron into the tissues.

Hemolysis : The disruption of the red cell membrane with the subsequent loss of cellular contents. Immune hemolysis is the result of the binding of complement on the cell membrane concurrent with the binding of antibody to a red cell antigen.

Hemolytic anemia : Anemia associated with the destruction (hemolysis) of red blood cells.

Hemolytic disease of the newborn (HDN): A disease characterized by the destruction of fetal/newborn red cells resulting from the placental transfer of maternal alloantibody.

Hemophilia A: An inherited sex-linked disorder characterized by low levels of Factor VIII-C activity.

Hemophilia-B: An inherited (sex-linked) disorder associated with a deficiency of Factor IX.

Hemosiderosis : Deposition of iron in tissues and organs which may result from the long-term administration of blood to patients with chronic anemia.

Hepatitis : Inflammation of the liver.

Hepatitis-A : The form of hepatitis generally transmitted by the fecal-oral route. Transmission of hepatitis A by transfusion is extremely rare.

Hepatitis-B : The form of hepatitis that is transmitted by transfusion. The incidence of hepatitis B has decreased with the advent of sensitive donor screening for the surface antigen (Hb, Ag).

Hepatitis-C : Before the viral genome was discovered, this disease was reerred to as non-A, non-B (NANB) hepatitis. Anti-HCV testing began in 1990 and has decreased the incidence of transfusion transmitted infection. Surrogate testing for HCV infection includes alanine aminotransaminase and anti-Hb.

Hepatitis-D : A hepatitis virus that as capable of causing disease only in the presence of hepatitis-B virus (HBV). Screening of blood for HBV results in a low risk of transfusion associated hepatitis-D infection.

Hereditary spherocytosis : An inherited disorder characterized by hemolysisi, spherocytosis, anemia, jaundice and splenomegaly.

Heterozygous : Referring to the condition in which two alleles for a given trait are different.

High-grade-D": A weakend expression of the D antigen associated with the inheritance of a C-producing gene on the opposite chromosome from a D-producing gene.

High incidence antigens : antigens that occur in greater than 99.9 per cent of the population.

High-protein reagents : Reagents that are enhanced by the additionof significant amounts of protein such as albumin. Such reagents are useful in the detection of IgG antibodies that may not agglutinate red cells suspended in saline media.

High-titer, low-avidity (HTLA) antibodies : A group of antibodies which react with characteristic fragile and weak agglutination, often characterized by high (usually greater than 1 : 64) titers.

Histamine : A substance produced from the amino acid histidine, the release of which results in increased gastric secretion, dilatationof capillaries, and contraction of bronchial smooth muscle.

HIV 1, 2 : HTLV-I/II : Viruses that have been documented to be transmitted by blood transfusion.

Homeostasis : That function of the immune system which removes efete or damaged self-components, such as aged red cells.

Homozygous : Pertaining to the condition in which the two alleles for a given trait are the same.

Human leukocyte antigens (HLA) : Glycoprotein antigens found on the surface of all nucleated cells of the body, including most circulating blood cells : lymphocytes, monocytes, granulocytes, and platelets.

Humoral immunity : Immunity mediated by antibodies.

Hybrid glycophorins : abnormal glycophorins resulting sialoglycoproteins, which causes the production of a number of unique low-incidence antigens in the MNSs system.

Hydrophobic : Insoluble in water.

Hydrops fetalis : a clinical condition in infants characterized by cardiac insufficiency with resultant edema and respiratory distress.

Hyperacute rejection : Rapid and extensive graft rejection associated with preformed HLA or ABO antibodies.

Hypersplenism : An enlarged spleen.

Hyperventilation : The increased inspiration and expiration of air which can result from an increase in either depth or rate of respiration. Hyperventilation results in carbon dioxide depletion with the associated fall in blood pressure, vasoconstriction, and sometimes syncope and is usually associated with anxiety.

Hypervolemia : Increased blood volume.

Hypoalbuminemia : Decreased serum albumin levels.

Hypoproteinemia : An abnormal decrease in the concentrations of protein in the blood.

Hypovolemia : A decrease in blood volume.

Hypoxemia : Insufficient oxygenation of the blood.

Hypoxia : Insuficient delivery of oxygen to the tissues.

Icterus gravis neonatorum : Jaundice of the newborn resulting from accelerated red cell destruction.

Idiopathic thrombocytopenic purpura : Abnormally low numbers of circulating platelets of unknown cause.

Immediate spin saline crossmatch : A compatibility test between donor red cells and recipient serum. The test is performed in a 0.9 per cent saline medium at room temperature and functions as a check for ABO compatibility. This abbreviated crossmatch can be performed if the recipient has no unexpected antibodies and no record of previous antibodies.

Immunodominant group : The portion of the epitope or antigenic determinant that binds most strongly with the antibody. The immunodominant group gives the antigen its specificity.

Immunodominant sugar : The terminal sugar that confers ABO antigen speci-ficity.

Immunogenicity : The degree to which an antigen is capable of eliciting an immune response.

Immunoglobulin : Any of the structurally related glycoproteins that function as antibodies. Immunoglobulins are divided into five classes based on their structure and function.

Incomplete dominance : The condition in which the products (traits) of both alleles are expressed but the effect of one allele is stronger than the other.

Increased osmotic fragility : Abnormal sensitivity of red cells to lysis in various concentrations of saline.

Indirect antiglobulin test (IAT) : A two-step test used to determine if antibody reacts with antigen on red blood cells in vitro.

Indirect or second-order exclusion : Exclusion of paternity because a child does not posses either of a pair of antigens possessed by the alleged father.

Informed consent : A process by which an individual is given necessary medical facts concerning inherent risks and signs a consent form authorizing the procedure and indicating that he or she understands the risks involved.

Inhibition (neutralization) : Inactivation of an antibody resulting from binding with soluble antigen. Blood group substances in saliva, for example, bind with their corresponding antibody, reducing the ability of the antibody to bind with particulate antigen (red cells).

Inhibitor (circulating anticoagulant): An endogenous substances in the blood which directly inhibits the activity of plasma coagulation factors.

Innate immunity : The nonspecific ability of the host to respond to injury or potential infection.

Intraoperative salvage : The process of collecting blood containing fluid from the surgical site. Blood thus collected can be reinfused through a suitable filter with or without subsequent processing.

Intrauterine transfusions : Treatment of fetal anemia by the transfusion of blood to the fetus. Blood can be infused into the peritoneal cavity, from which it is absorbed by the fetus, or can be administered directly into the umbilical vein.

Intravascular hemolysis : The destruction of transfused red cells within the vascular compartment, due to either immunologic or nonimmunologic means. Immune intravascular hemolysis is commonly associated with the transfusion of ABO-incompatible red cells.

Intravenous immune gamma globulin : A modified gamma globulin fraction that is safc for intravenous infusion.

Ischemia : Local deficiency in blood supply to an organ or tissue.

Isoelectric focussing (IEF) : A procedure used to further subtype serologically defined antigens by identifying protein isoelectric points, thus determining amino acid composition.

Isotype switching : A switch from IgM to IgG secretion by B cells.

Joint Commission for the Accreditation of Healthcare Organization (JCAHO) The organization that develops standards for health care delivery and provides a voluntary inspection and accreditation program for hospitals and other health care delivery units.

Kernicterus : A grave condition resulting from the passage of bilirubin into the brain and spinal cord.

Kleihauer-Berke stain : A technique used to quantitate fetal-maternal hemorrhage based on the fact that fetal hemoglobin is resistant to acid elution, whereas adult hemoglobin is not. Estimates of fetal bleed are made from counts of fetal cells per 1000 adult cells in a sample of maternal blood.

K (Kellnull) : Resulting from the inheritance of two K° genes and associated with red cells that lack all Kell system antigens but do express large amounts of K_4 antigen.

Lacto-N-neotetraosylceramide : The precursor substance for the Le antigen in plasma.

Lacto-N-tetrose : The precursor substance for the Le antigen in body fluids.

Lectin : Any of a group of plant substances capable of binding specifically with antigen substances (sugars) on the surface of red blood cells, resulting in agglutination. Dolichos bifloris, for example, is a lectin with anti-A_1 specificity.

Leukoagglutinins : Antibodies to antigens on the surface of white cells that can be identified by their ability to agglutinate antigen-positive cells.

Leukocyte-poor red blood cells : A red cell component from which white cells have been removed by one of a number of leukodepletion methods, including sedimentation, centrifugation, washing, or filtration. This component is useful for patients who have exhibited severe febrile reactions. Refer to leukocyte reduction.

Leukocyte reduction filters (third-generation): Adhesion filters that effectively remove 99.0 to 99.9 pe rcent of the leukocytes. These filters can be used for the filtration of both red cells and platelets.

Leukocyte reduction : removal of 70 to 99 per cent of the original leukocytes in aunit of red cells.

Lewis antigens : Soluble antigens that are adsorbed onto the red cell surface and are not an integral part of the red cell membrane.

Linkage : The location of genes in close proximity on a chromosome.

Linkage disequilibrium : The occurrence of a haplotype in the population more frequently than would be expected by probability.

LISS-Polybrene : The combination of low ionic strength saline and Polybrene, which is capable of bringing about the agglutination of red cells.

Lookback : A process by which all recipients of blood and blood products from an HIV-positive donor are identified and informed of the possible risks associated with these products.

Low grade D": A weakened expression of the D-antigen associated with a genetically transmitted D".

Low-incidence antigens : Antigens that occur in less tha 1 per cent of the population.

Low-ionic polycation tests : The combination of red cells antibody uptake in a low ionic strength, low-pH medium and the use of a chemical red cell aggregating agent. If antibody has coated the cells, the aggregation does not disperse.

Low ionic strength saline (LISS) : A blood banking reagent that potentiates some antigen-antibody reactions by lowering the ionic strength and thus decreasing the net charge of red cells.

Low-protein reagents : Reagents that are not enhanced by the addition of protein. These are frequently termed saline reagents.

L/S ratio : Levels of two phospholipid surfactants found in the amniotic fluid. As the fetal lung matures, the lecithin levels (L) increase and the sphingomyelin (S) remains constant. An L/S ratio of greater than 2.0 is a good predictor of fetal lung maturity.

Lymphokines : A general term for those soluble mediators of the immune response other than complement and antibody which are secreted by sensitized lymphocytes upon contact with antibody.

Macrophage clearance : The ability of macrophages to remove antibody-coated cells via the Fc receptor.

Major crossmatch : A procedure used to determine compatibility between the red cells of the donor and the serum (plasma) of the recipient.

Major histocompatibility complex restriction : The control of a vivo immune responses by HLA antigen expression.

Malaria/babesiosis : Protozoan diseases transmitted by transfusion. Both are rare and no donor testing is available.

Maximum surgical blood order schedule (MSBOS) : Criteria developed from institutional usage statistics providing a figure for the number of units to be crossmatched for any given surgical procedure.

Meiosis : Cell division and replication which result in the formation of haploid gametes (eggs and sperm), which carry either the maternal or paternal genetic information.

McLeod phenotype : A phenotype associated with a decreased expression of Kell antigens on red cells. McLeod phenotype is associated with a pathologic process known as the McLeod syndrome, which is characterized by anemia and neuromuscular disorders.

McLeod syndrome : The pathologic process usually associated with the McLeod phenotype, which includes hematologic, cardiac, and neurologic defects.

Meconium : the first stool produced by a newborn.

Microaggregate filters (second-generation) : Screen or depth type filters that remove aggregates smaller than 170 microns. Microaggregate screen filters have pore sizes ranging from 20 to 40 microns and effectively remove 70 to 90 per cent of the leukocytes.

Microlymphocytotoxicity tests : Tests used to screen for and identify HLA antigen/antibody reactions using complement fixation and cell lysis as end points.

Microplate methods : serologic procedures that use micro-well plates rather than test tubes.

Microscopic examination : The observation of agglutination reactions with the aid of the low power objective of the microscope. One should always check manufacturer's directions and institutional protocols to determine if microscopic reading is appropriate for the test being performed.

Miltenberger system : A subsystem of the MNSs system producing anumber of low-incidence antigens.

Minor crossmatch : A procedure used to determine compatibility between the serum (plasma) of the donor and the red cells of the recipient. This test is no longer used routinely but has historical significance.

Mitosis : Cell division and replication which result in the formation of two diploid daughter cells with exactly the same genetic information as the parent cell.

Mixed field agglutination : The agglutination pattern in which some cells are aggluinated whereas others ae not. Mixed field agglutination is most frequently associated with serologic testing in which there are two or more cell populations, such as a recently transfused patient.

Mixed lymphocyte culture (MLC) : A serologic assay used to determine Class II compatibility between a donor and recipient by measuring the incorporationof radiolabeled marker as an indicator of blast transformation.

Monoclonal reagents : Reagents produced by hybridization techniques.

Monocytes : Phagocytic leukocytes produced in the bone marrow. Monocyte are transported to the tissues, such as lung, liver, and spleen, where they develop into macrophages.

Mosaic : A complex antigen, such as D, that has more than a single antigenic determinant.

N-acetylgalactosaminyltransferase : An enzyme that transfers the sugar N-acetylgalactosamine (GalNAc) to the H antigen, conferring group A specificity.

National Committee for Clinical Laboratory Standards (NCCLS): An organization that provides published standards for clinical laboratory science in all areas of practice, such as a standard format for procedures manuals.

Neocytes : A population of relatively young red cells. Larger and less dense younger red cells can be separated from older red cells that are smaller and more dense by differential centrifugation techniques. During automated cell washing theyoung cells are pushed out of the bag earlier and collected for transfusion.

Neonate : An infant less than 4 months of age.

Neutropenia : A decrease in the number of circulating neutrophils in the peripheral blood.

Nonhemolytic febrile trnasfusion reactions : Fever responses due to the transfusion of HLA-incompatible leukocytes. These reactions can be associated with the transfusion of any component containing residual donor white cells and can be reduced by teh use of bedside leukofiltration.

Null cells : The population of lymphocytes that carry neither T-nor B-cell markers. Natural killer (NK) cells are part of this group of cells.

Oligonucleotide probes, polymerase chain reaction (PCR), and direct nucleotide sequencing: Method of gene analysis useful in the identification and subtyping of HLA antigens.

Oncotic pressure : The pressure exerted by colloids in solution. This pressure affects the balance of fluid in the intravascular and extravascular spaces. Decreases in blood protein (colloid) result in the movement of water out of the vascular compartment and into the extravascular spaces, resulting in edema. Increases in intravascular oncotic pressure (as with the infusion of 25 per cent albumin) results in the movement of water into the vascular compartment.

Optical aids : Devices that enhance the reading of test tube agglutination reactions.

Orthopnea : Difficulty breathing in any but in an erect position.

Oxygen-carrying capacity : The relative ability of red blood cells to combine with oxygen and release the bound oxygen to tissues.

Oxygen dissociation curve : The sigmoid relationship between PO_2 and O_2 saturation of hemoglobin. The P_{50} in the PO_2 at which hemoglobin is 50 per cent saturated.

Pancytopenia : Decreased numbers of all blood cell lines.

Parabens : Substances added to preserve reagents which may result in some discrepant serologic results.

Passive transfer : Antibody not actively produced by the host. Such antibodies can be acquired by the transfer of maternal antibody across the placenta or the administration of antibody in the plasma portion of blood/components.

Paternity index : The genetic odds in favour of paternity calculated from the phenotypes of the other, alleged father, and offspring.

Pedigree chart : A diagrammatic method of illustrating the inheritance of genes within a given family.

Percutaneous : Application of substances through the skin either by friction or by injection.

Perioperative hemodilution (isovolemic): The exchange of blood for plasma substitutes such as normal saline which effectively reduces the hematoccit while maintaining normal blood volume.

Phenotype : Inherited traits that are expressed in an individual.

Phototherapy : The use of light to degrade bilirubin in mildly jaundiced infants.

Physician peer review (transfusion commitee) : The process by which physicians review transfusion practice within the institution using a set of predetermined criteria. The goal of peer review is improvement in the quality of blood transfuion practice.

Platelet concentrates : A blood component prepared by centrifugation from aunit of donor blood prior to refrigeration. Platelets are indicated for patients who are at risk of hemorrhage or who are bleeding secondary to low platelet number of dysfunctional platelets.

Plateletpheresis : Collection of platelets by cytapheresis. The pheresis methodology allows for large platelet yields from a single donor, which makes this product valuable for the patient who requires HLA-matched platelets.

Pluripotential cell : A bone marrow cell, that is capable of differentiation into many different cll types.

Polyagglutination : Red cells that are agglutinated by a large percentage of human sera regardless of blood types but not agglutinated by autologous serum. Most forms of polyagglutination are due to the exposure of some hidden receptor on the surface of the red cell.

Polyethylene glycol (PEG) : A commercially availableenhancement reagent used for the detection and identification of weak IgG antibodies.

Polyhydramnios : An excessive amount of amniotic fluid.

Polymorphic : Pertaining to the existence of two or more phenotypes in a population.

Polymorphism : The quality of having many different forms or states. In the science of genetics, they refers to many different phenotypes.

Pooled products : Pooling of multiple units of components (e.g platelets or cryoprecipitate) into one bag for ease of transfusion.

Portal hypertension : Increased pressure int he protal vein, which delivers blood to the liver. This is commonly due to some obstruction of blood flow through the liver.

Postoperative blood salvage : The process of collecting blood-containing fluid from a closed site such as chest tube drainage.

Postpartum : after delivery

Post-transfusion purpura (PTP) : Red discoloration of the skin caused by hemorrhage, resulting from immune destruction transfused platelets by antiplatelet antibodies in the recipient.

Postzone : The condition of antibody excess in which few agglutinates form.

Predeposit donation : The donation of one or more units of blood by a donor for his or her own use for some anticipated future need such as pending surgery.

Primed lymphocyte test (PLT) : A serologic assay that uses previously primed responder cells in a mixed lymphocyte culture text so that results can be obtained more rapidly.

Private epitopes : Antigenic deterninants that are the product of a single gene.

Proband/propositus : The individual with a certain disease or other inherited trait of interest.

Progenitor cell (stem cell) : A cell that gives rise to a specific cell type during hematopoiesis.

Prozone : The condition of antigen excess in which few agglutinates form.

Public epitopes : Antigenic determinants that are produced by more than one gene.

Pulmonary edema : An accumulation of fluid in the lungs.

Pulse pressure : The difference between the diastolic and systolic pressures. The systolic pressure is normally approximately 40 mm Hg greater than the diastolic.

P value of 0.05 : A probability of 5 per cent or less than the phenomenon occurred by chance, also known as 95 per cent confidence limits.

recessiveness : Inheritance in which a trait is expressed only when the allele is present in the homozygous form.

Red blood cells/packed cells : The blood component prepared by removing most of the residual plasma (200 to 250 mL) from a unit of centrifuged or sedimented whole blood. Red blood cells have the same red cell volume and therefore the same oxygen-carrying capacity as whole blood in a significantly reduced volume. Red cells are indicated for the treatment of anemia in normovolemic patients.

Refractory : Exhibiting general unresponsiveness to therapy. Patients who do not respond to platelet transfusion with the expected increase in platelet number are termed refractory.

Regulator type RHnull : A phenotype resulting from the inheritance of two X°r genes.

Rejuvenated red cells : Red cells produced by the addition of agents capable of restoring concentrations of ATP and 2,3-DPG in stored red cell products. Adequate levels of ATP are necessary for red blood cell viability, and 2, 3-DPG is necessary for satisfactory oxygen delivery to tissues.

Responders : Individuals who produce antibody when stimulated by foreign antigen.

Restriction fragment length polymorphism (RELP) : A molecular typing technique used to study Class II antigenes.

reticulocytosis : An increase of immature red cells (reticulocytes) in the circulation.

Reticuloendothelial system (RES)/mononuclear phagocytic system (MPS) : A group of cells having in common the ability to sequester inert particles, vital dyes, etc. Included in this system are the fibroblasts of the bone marrow; macrophages, endothelial linings of the liver, spleen, and bone marrow, and reticular cells of the lymphatic system.

Retinitis pigmentosa : An inherited condition associated with the progressive loss of retinal response.

Rh control reagent : The manufacturer's control that contains all of the components of the anti-D reagent except for the antibody. This reagent serves as a negative control for Rh typing.

Rh immune globulin (RhIG): A solutiono f gamma globulin containing anti-D. A 300 μg dose of RhIg, if administered within 72 hours of delivery, protects against alloimmunization of the mother to the D antigen of the fetus. Each vial of 300 μg of RhIG protects against 30 mL of fetal whole blood or 15 mL of packed cells.

Rhnull phenotype : An inherited characteristic in which none of the Rh antigens is expressed.

Ringer's lactate (Ringer's lactated solution) : An intravenous fluid containing sodium chloride, potassium chloride, calcium chloride, and sodium lactate in water. The solution is used to replace volume and electrolytes, but because it contains calcium, it should not be added to blood/components.

Resetting test : A screening test for fetal-maternal hemorrhage. The test is based on the principle that Rh-positive fetal cells coated with anti-D form rosettes with Rh-positive indicator cells, making them distinguishable from the Rh-negative maternal cell population.

Rouleaux : Red cell rolls that have the appearance of a stack of coins.

Rule-out cells : Cells on the panel which do not react with the antibody being identified and can be used to eliminate possible solutions.

Saline replacement techniques : Replacement of serum with saline at the final stage of a test in order to disperse interfering rouleaux.

Saline Rh reagents : A synonym for low-protein reagents.

Saline test system : An in vitro test procedure that uses a normal (0.9 per cent NaCl) saline medium. This system is often used to detect IgM antibodies.

0.9 per cent saline (normal saline) : a volume expander that is compatible with red blood cells.

Satellite bag : Additional bag attached to the main donor set by sterile tubin. These satellite bags are used for the removal of various blood components, avoiding nonsterile entry of the system.

Secretor : An individual who has inherited at least one Se gene which results in the secretion of ABH antigens into the body fluids. These individuals make up approximately 80 per cent of the random population.

Segments : Sealed portions of the integral donor tubing which lead from the collection bag to the needle during phlebotomy. Segments contain small aliquots of donor blood which can be used for pretransfusion testing.

Sensitization : The binding of antibody or complement components to a red cell antigen.

Septicemia : A serious condition marked by the presence of pathologic microorganisms in the blood.

Serologically defined : Refers to HLA antigens that can be identified by the microlymphocytotoxicity test (HLA-A, HLA-B, HLA-C, HLA-Dr, and HLA-DQ).

Serotonin : The chemical 5-hydroxytryptamine, a potent vasoconstrictor.

Sex (X)-linked inheritance : Inheritance by means of an allele carried on the X-chromosome.

Shock : A syndrome associated with insufficient return of blood to the heart for normal function and subsequent diminished blood flow to vital tissues.

Siderophore : A cell or a substane that has an affinity for iron.

Single donor plasma and cryoprecipitate poor plasma : Components that lack labile coagulation factors but contain stable coagulation factors.

Single donor plasma, liquid plasma : The product prepared by the separation of plasma from whole blood before the fifth day after expiration. When stored in the frozen state at- 18°C, the product can be kept for up to 5 years and is known as plasma.

Single donor screening cells : Cells from individual group O donors selected for their antigen typing configuration. Sets of two or three such cells are selected to screen for most of the commonly encountered red cell alloantibodies and are used for routine antibody detection.

Specificity : The configuration of an antibody which results in its reaction only with the unique antigenic determinant that elicited its response.

Sphygmomanometers : Blood pressure measurement devices with inflatable pressurized cuffs.

Splenomegaly : An enlarged spleen.

Splits.subtypes : HLA antigens may have additional epitopes that divided them into one or more subtypes (splits); for example, HLA-A10 has two splits, HLA-A25 and HLA-A26. Both of these splits are positive for the HLA-A10 antigen.

Standard blood filters (first-generation): Screen filters with a pore size of 170 to 260 microns. These filters are required for all blood/component therapy and have the ability to screen out large debris such as fibrin clots.

Sterile connection (docking) device : An instrument capable of heat welding plastic tubing in a sterile manner, often used when blood components are needed and satellite bags are not available.

Stomatocytes : Red cells with a slit-shaped rather than a circular zone of central pallor.

Storage lesion : Biochemical changes that take place in blood during storage.

Suppressor gene : A gene that diminshes the effect of another independently inherited gene.

Surrogate test : A laboratory test that indirectly screens for an infectious disease.

surveillance : That function of the immune system which detects and destroys mutant cells, thus providing protection from malignancy.

Survival studies : Measurement of the in vivo survival of radiolabeled red cells. This technique is useful in determining the potential survival of donor red cells in a recipient's circulation.

Symptomatic anemia : A condition in which there is a decrease in the number of the circulating red cells, the amount of hemoglobin, or the volume of packed red cells per volume of blood. When anemia is severe enough, a patient presents with some or all of the following symptoms: pallor, weakness, vertigo, headache, sore tongue, drowsiness, malaise, dyspnea, tachycardia, palpitation, angina pectoris, gastrointestinal disturbances, amenorrhea, and slight fever.

Syphilis : A sexually transmitted disease that is rarely transmitted by the transfusion of blood that has been stored more than 72 hours. Serologic testing for syphilis is performed on donor blood.

Systolic pressure : The period of more pressue in the arterial system which corresponds to the time in the heart cycle in which the muscle contracts and expels its contents (systole).

T lymphocytes (T cells) : T-lymphocytes, or thymus-dependent lymphocytes, originate from lymphoid stem cells, differentiate under the influence of thymus hormones, are characterized by cell surface antigens, and are primarily responsible for cell-mediated immunity.

Teratogen : A substance that causes the abnormal development of the fetus.

Thalassemia : An inherited anemia caused by the production of abnormal hemoglobin molecules.

Therapeutic apheresis : Application of apheresis procedures to the treatment of disease.

Thiol (sulfhydryl) reagents : Substances that cleave the disulfide bonds of IgM molecules, abolishing the ability of the molecule to agglutinate or bind complement. Thiol reagents (DTT and 2-ME) are useful in differentiating IgM antibodies from IgG antibodies.

Thrombocytopathy : A condition of functionally abnormal platelets.

Thrombocytopenia : Decreased platelet number.

Thrombogenic : A tendency to cause blood clots or thrombi.

Thrombotic thrombocytopenic purpura (TTP) : A disorder characterized by decreased platelet numbers, hemolytic anemia, and thrombosis.

Titer : The highest dilution at which agglutination can be detected.

Titration : A technique involving the serial dilution of an antiserum to determine the range of antibody activity (titer). In a mixture of antibodies, specificities can sometimes be distinguished using titration methods.

Transferases : Enzymes that transfer chemical groups from one compound to another. A and B gene products are glucosyltransferases, meaning that they transfer sugars. These sugars are responsible for ABO blood group specificity.

Transfusion-associated graft-versus-host disease (TA-GVHD) : Proliferation o f immunologically competent donor cells in an immunocompromised recipient. Also at risk are individuals who receive blood and components from blood relatives. Such reactions can be avoided by irradiation fo blood and components that contain white cells.

Transfusion reaction : Any adverse outcome associated with the infusion of blood or blood components.

Transfusion-related acute lung injury (TRALI) : Pulmonary edema, not associated with left heart failure, that is usually due to the transfusion of preformed donor leukoagglutinins in the plasma of blood components.

Transfusion service : A facility that is traditionally housed in the institution where transfusion takes place, usually a hospital. The role of the transfusion service is to provide the necessary testing and support to ensure the appropriate and safe transfusion of blood, blood components, and blood products, including pretransfusion testing, antibody identification, product selection, and monitoring of transfusion outcomes.

Two-stages enzyme test : A test in which red cells are pretreated with proteolytic enzymes for use in antibody identification/confirmation tests. Some antibodies react more strongly with enzyme treated cells, whereas some antigens are destroyed and thereby the reactions diminished.

Type and screen : Abbreviated compatibility testing that does not include a crossmatch. Such procedures are recommended for patients with a low probability of transfusion.

Type-I and II structures : Precursor substances and antigens in the ABO system differentiated by the type linkage between terminal carbohydrates.

Ultrasonography : Using high-frequency sound waves (approx. 20,000 cycles per second) to produce an image of an organ or tissue based on the fact that ultrasound waves move at different velocities in tissues of differing elasticity and density.

Unexpected antibodies : Red cell antibodies that, unlike the naturally occurring anti-A or anti-B, are not routinely present in the serum and are generally a result of red cell stimulation (transfusion or pregnancy).

Universal precautions : Guidelines based on the assumption that all body fluids are equally capable of transmitting infectious disease, and, therefore, the same level of precaution is used with all specimens.

Urticaria : hives.

Vasovagal syncope : Sudden fainting due to hypotension resulting from nervous system response to stress or trauma.

Vernix : The deposit that covers the fetus during intra-uterine life.

von Willebrand's disease : An inherited disorder characterized by decreased levels of Factors VIII-C, VIII : vWF, and VIII : ag.

Warfarin sodium : The generic name for 3-(αacetonyl-benzyl) 4-hydroxycoumarin, an anticoagulant drug that acts by inhibiting the synthesis of the vitamin K-dependent factors (II, VII, IX and X). Product names include Coumarin. Panwarfin, and Sofarin.

Washed red blood cells : Red cells that have been subjected to serial washing and centrifugation processes in order to remove platelets, plasma, and most of the white blood cells.

Wharton's jelly : A gelatinous substance from the umbilical cord which is rich in hyaluronic acid. This substance can contaminate cord blood specimens and interfere with serologic testing.

Whole blood : The source product for all blood components production which consists of red cells, white cells, platelets, and plasma collected into an approved anticoagulant/preservative solution. A unit of whole blood has a volume of 450 ± 45 mL. Whole blood is indicated for hypovolemic patients with clinical symptoms associated with poor oxygen-carrying capacity.

Whole blood, modified : Whole blood from which cryoprecipitate and/or platelets have been removed.

Window period : that period between infection and the ability to detect disease through laboratory testing.

ZZAP : a mixture of cysteine-activated papain and dithiothreitol. Treatment of cells with ZZAP removes the activity of a number of blood group antigens. The technique is useful for the preparation of artificial K cells.

ANNEXURES

ANNEXURE - I

Offences and penalties as laid down under the drugs and cosmetics ACT, 1940 and rules there under concerning blood banks

	Offence	Penalty
1.	Manufacture for sale or selling Whole Human Blood I.P. without valid licence as required under clause (C) of u/s 18.	Imprisonment for a term which shall not be less than one year but which may extend to three years and with fine which shall not be less than five thousand rupees, u/s 27 (b) (ii) of the Act.
2.	Manufacture for sale or selling Whole Human Blood I.P. contaminated with Human I virus (HIV) or Hepatitis B. Virus or Not sterile is a sub-standard drug within meaning of 16 (i) (a) of the Act.	Imprisonment for a term which shall not be less than five years but which may extended to a term of life and with fine, which shall not be less than ten thousand rupees u/s 27 (a). Because the Whole Human Blood I.P. contaminated with human Immuno Deficiency Virus or Hepatitis Virus is likely to cause death or is likely to cause such harm as would amount to grievous hurt, within the meaning of Section 320, IPC.
3.	Manufacture of Whole Human Blod I.P. for sale or selling which is not labelled in prescribed manner is misbranded within the meaning of Section 17(b) of the Act.	Imprisoment for a term which shall not be less than one year but which may extend to 2 years and with fine of Rupees ten thousand u/s 27(d) of the Act.
4.	Manufacture of Whole Human Blood I.P. for sale or selling not in accordance with the conditions of licence issued for such purpose.	Imprisonment for a term which shall not be less than one year but which may extend to 2 years and with fine under Section 27(d) of the Act.

ANNEXURE - II

Offences and Penalties under Drugs and Cosmetics Act and Rules Regarding Blood Banks

	Offence	*Penality*
1.	Manfacture for sale adulterated/spurious drug which is likely to cause death or grievious hurt	Imprisonment not less than 5 years, may extend to life imprisonment and fine not less Rs. 10,000/- Section 27(b) (i).
2.	Adulterated drug not covered by above Section 27 (b) (ii)	Imprisonment not less than one year, may extend to 3 years and fine and less than Rs. 5000/-. Court may impose lesser punishment with reason recorded.
3.	Manufacture of drug without valid licence. Section 27(b)(i).	Imprisoonment not less than one year, may extend to 3 years and fine not less than Rs. 5000/-Court may impose lesser punish ment with reason recorded.
4.	Spurious drugs not covered by (i) above Sec-27(c)	Imprisonment not less than 3 years which may extend to 5 years with fine not less than Rs. 5000/- .Court may impose lesser punishment but not less than one year imprisonment with reasons recorded.
5.	Drug manufactured in contravention of any other provision of the Act or Rules (Section 29 (d).	Imprisonment not less than one year which may extend to 2 years with fine. Court may impose lesser punishment not less than one year imprisonment with reasons recorded.
6.	Non-disclosure of the information regarding manufacturer etc. and not keeping the documents (Sec 28 & 28-A).	Imprisonment for one year or with fine upto Rs. 1000/- or both.
7.	Subsequent offences for (i) & (ii)	Imprisonment for a term not less than 2 years which may extend to six years and with a fine not less than Rs. 10,000/-. Court may impose lesser punishment with reasons recorded.

(contd.)

ANNEXURE - II

Offences and Penalities under Drugs and Cosmetics Act and Rules Regarding Blood Banks (Contd...)

	Offence	*Penality*
8.	Subsequent offences for (iii)	Imprisonment for a term not less than 6 years which may extend to 10 years and fine not less than Rs. 10,000/-
9.	Subsequent offences for (iv)	Imprisonment not less than 2 years which may extend to 4 years with fine not less than Rs. 5000/- or both

Cognizance of offences :

a) Only an inspector or a person aggreived or a recognised Consumer Association can institute prosecution.

b) Only a court not inferior than first class Judicial Magistrate or Metropolitan Magistrate shall try the offence.

c) There is no provision under Drugs and Cosmetics Act and Rules for trying a doctor for using blood which is free from infection and transfusing to a patient.